CHARMING LACHESIS
An Impression of Modern Medicine

Joseph T. Batuello, MD, JD

Copyright © 2012 Joseph T. Batuello

All rights reserved.

ISBN: 1470074710
ISBN-13: 978-170074715

LCCN:

DEDICATION

To all of those who are determined to live life to its fullest, regardless of their circumstances.

CONTENTS

	Acknowledgments	i
	Preface	iii
1	Lachesis: The Genesis of Medicine	1
2	Disease	18
3	Diagnosis	41
4	Therapy	60
5	Ethics	84
6	The Business of Medicine	114
7	The Modern Practice of Medicine	153
8	Atropos: The End	179
	Bibliography	191

ACKNOWLEDGMENTS

I would like to thank Alan Fine, MD for his patience during many hours of conversation regarding the subject of this book, for his review of the manuscript and many thoughtful suggestions. I am also grateful to Andrew Sullivan, MD for his thoughts and insights regarding medicine and end-of-life care.

PREFACE

The premise of this book is that it is possible to learn many of the important things in life through observation and experience. It is certainly possible to learn timeless truths by studying and contemplating the works of classical philosophers, writers and thinkers, but is also possible to appreciate such truths by observing the commonplace and humdrum in our everyday lives. There is much wisdom and understanding to be gained from raising one's children or dedicating oneself to mastering a trade. There is much we can learn from little pleasures and little annoyances. Life is full of lessons that are accessible to the curious, the observant and the adventurous. This book attempts to make use of this notion to describe modern medicine, not by rigorously detailing its historical development or analyzing its philosophical principles, but by simply trying to explain how it appears from the vantage of everyday life.

This book is not meant to be a thorough analysis or exhaustive description of any of the subjects found within it. It is intended neither as a critique, nor as a primer. There is no attempt to cover either the breadth or depth of the subject. This book does not attempt to make an argument although, as with any impression, it cannot be completely independent of a perspective. The purpose of this book is not to identify a problem and propose a remedy, rather it is meant to convey a set of impressions that result from particular experiences and specific observations.

The impressionist school of art took its name from the painting *Impression, soleil levant*, or *Impression, sunrise* by Claude Monet. The painting conveyed certain aspects of a sunrise without looking exactly like one. A similar ambition is responsible for the form of this book: the intent is not to convey objective description as much as to provide a combination of perceptions that is recognizable, even for want of detail. As a result, the form of the book reflects the nature of its subject matter, in that much of medicine consists of forming impressions from fragmentary observations, remote experiences and convenient perspectives. When a radiologist examines an x-ray, it is for the purpose of interpreting it, rather than merely describing it. The intent of this book is to present various observations and thoughts about healthcare with the idea that the reader's interpretation of them will not be limited by cold, objective description.

There are several concepts that recur throughout the discussions in this book: that human beings are tool users, that competing interests are inherent in medicine, and that many of the characteristics of modern medicine, both the good and the bad, are rational. These concepts are taken as points of reference for some of the discussions that follow, and are taken as valid simply because they are readily observed throughout everyday life. They are among those basic and fundamental elements that hopefully will combine to convey an impression of modern medicine.

While the perspective of this book is influenced heavily by experience with western, scientifically based medicine, there is no intended implication as to the validity of other healthcare disciplines or traditions. Modern medicine consists largely of western medicine, and so observations about medicine will mostly originate from there. To the extent that there are some truths that apply to all healing disciplines, it is hoped that this unavoidable point of reference will not obscure them.

This book is not intended as a philosophy of medicine, but it does try to apply some philosophical methods. There is an attempt to identify some of the essentials of disease, diagnosis and therapy, and to note the influence of business, ethics and cultural forces that shape the way medicine is practiced. If the reader can perceive any of his or her own experience in the chapters that follow, this book will have achieved its aim.

Joseph T. Batuello

1

LACHESIS
THE GENESIS OF MODERN MEDICINE

Everybody dies. This deduction follows readily from the vast majority of human history. It has always been possible to identify some date in the relatively recent past, whereby all persons born before that date eventually died, and that date is constantly changing, always proceeding forward in time. History also allows one to conclude that nearly everyone who dies will die of disease or trauma. There may some definitional quibbling as to whether freezing to death or drug overdoses or carbon monoxide poisoning conforms to this generalization, but experience suggests that an individual's demise will be due to an identifiable infirmity or injury.

The ancient Greeks, or some of them anyway, referred to the mythological Fates, or Moirae, who determined the span of an individual's life. These three female deities, Clotho, Lachesis, and Atropos, determined the length of the metaphorical thread of life, and thus the lifespan of every individual human. Clotho spun the thread of life from her distaff onto her spinning wheel; Lachesis measured out the length of thread, and thus the number of days of which each life would consist; and Atropos cut the thread at the critical point. The concept of the three Fates demonstrates that, while the ancient Greeks may have had individual ambitions and plans, there were some highly important details about life that were largely out of their hands.

The concept of the Fates may have helped the Greeks come to grips with the inevitability of death, and provided a measure of understanding as to why some lives ended with much unfilled promise. The Greeks however, like most other people, were not accepting of the notion that matters of disease and injury were necessarily left to deific whimsy. If Clotho could not be dissuaded from spinning or Atropos from cutting, perhaps Lachesis could be charmed into allowing a little greater length.

Although the ancient Greeks enshrined the Fates as part of their mythology, they did not concede that matters of life and death were completely out of their own hands. A great many ancient Greeks are remembered to history as physicians. Hippocrates is probably the most familiar to modernity, but others such as Androcydes, Soranus, and Diocles of Carystus, among many others, are remembered in history as prominent men of medicine. Greek physicians cared for the ill and injured, wrote treatises and texts spanning the scientific and mystical aspects of healing, and conducted investigations and made empirical observations about health and disease.

We know a fair amount about ancient Greek medicine because of the impressive historical record that the ancient Greeks created and passed on. While the Greeks certainly deserve recognition because of their surviving historical record, we may safely assume that the practice of medicine is not unique to any culture or civilization. No one invented medicine. Medicine existed wherever humans existed.

All civilizations of which we have record, and some that we know only through archeological discoveries, had beliefs and practices that we can recognize as the art, and now and then, the science of medicine. Native American, Chinese, African, Persian and Indian peoples all had theories regarding health and illness, remedies for various ailments, and traditions and customs for preserving their medical wisdom.

In 1991, hikers in the Tyrolean Alps discovered the frozen body of a man who had died approximately 5300 years prior. Among the possessions discovered along with the body was a crude medical kit containing birch mushrooms, a fungus confirmed to have antibacterial properties. In addition, the man's body bore tattoos that modern scientists think might have been related to a medical procedure similar to acupuncture. The precise source of the ancient Tyrolean's medical knowledge is unknown, but our remote ancestors appear to have engaged in medicinal practices that developed from such basic processes as observation, trial and error, and perhaps intuition.

Healing arts are intrinsic to humans because of the human capacity for higher cognition and the basic instincts common to complex species. Even animals engage in basic activities that serve a salutary purpose, such as licking wounds, seeking refuges in which to convalesce and avoiding use of injured limbs. Human beings however are tool users by nature. We use whatever is useful to accomplish a desired purpose, and develop those tools through constant improvement, observation and ingenuity. Simple observation makes it quite reasonable to use a tourniquet or bandage to control bleeding from a wound, or notice that parts of various plants have desirable effects in certain disease states. Human progress is enabled by the capacity to reason, inquire and model. Humans are curious by nature, and the great mysteries of disease, death, and suffering provide endless opportunities for contemplation and investigation.

One might also conjecture that humans' unique awareness of their own mortality and inherent fascination with spiritual and mystical aspects of living motivate them to seek interventions against death and disease. As was true for our ancestors, and no less so for us, disease, injury, suffering and death are ubiquitous experiences, and seeking some measure of control over such life-altering realities is both an instinctive and rational endeavor.

Human beings, through simple observation, cannot but notice the effects of diseases and bodily misfortune on their lives, ambitions and beliefs. They need only notice the ravages of plagues, or the trial of pregnancy that was mooted by early death of the infant, or death of the mother in childbirth. Even in the absence of such poignant experiences, human beings would make more basic observations such as that being sick made them feel bad, a condition that they would seek to avoid or ameliorate through some intervention. In a similar manner, parents are motivated by instincts to care for and nurture their offspring, to comfort them and relieve their suffering. It is quite natural to employ human ingenuity to these same ends. Medicine is the result of humankind's ability to perceive and contemplate the realities of existence as complex biological beings, and to use reason in search of a better life.

Human beings have the capacity to inquire into the nature of illness and trauma on the very large scale by, for example, observing the course and effects of epidemics. They may also do so on smaller scales by investigating the effects of remedies, identifying pathogens, and hypothesizing about the causes and cures of various diseases. When George Washington assumed command of the Continental Army, one of his challenges was to lessen the risk that his forces would be devastated by disease. Epidemics had been common in colonial America, and to minimize the chance that the prevailing patriotic fervor and love of liberty would be frustrated by cholera or small pox, Washington ordered a number of general health measures for his troops. These ranged from a program of the then-developing practice of smallpox inoculations, to more draconian policies such as having sentries shoot soldiers who urinated on the ground at Valley Forge. These interventions were dramatically effective. What General Washington had embraced were public health measures, rational responses to the epidemics and plagues associated with improved transportation, people concentrating into cities, and soldiers clustering in camps.

Public health interventions are not new. Many of the religious dietary laws, such as avoidance of pork and the attendant risk of trichinosis, had public health benefits. Innovations such as sanitation, quarantines, and early forms of vaccination were efforts to lessen the burden of certain communicable diseases by keeping people from contracting them in the first place. It is highly unlikely that the threat of smallpox that concerned General Washington could have been effectively addressed by simply treating those already infected. Even today, we can observe the dramatic effects that public health and disease eradication efforts have on life expectancy and other metrics of human health. It seems at least reasonable to believe that preventing disease across a broad population has a greater effect on average life spans than does treating disease individually after affliction. This is particularly obvious when considering diseases such as the acquired immunodeficiency syndrome, which for millions of persons infected early in the course of the epidemic had no effective treatment. The same principle applies to other diseases like hanta virus infection or meningococcal meningitis, for which treatments are often unsuccessful.

Smallpox was largely eradicated by public health measures, an outcome that would have been unobtainable by treating patients one-at-a-time. Nonetheless, the practice of medicine in which an individual practitioner treats an individual patient has developed continually throughout human history. Like most institutions that have survived for centuries or millennia, medicine endures because human beings have found it beneficial.

The benefits of medicine might be surmised to accrue to the human species as a whole, as in providing a survival advantage; to discrete societies or communities, such that ill health of individuals not impair their contributions of labor or talent; or to the individuals themselves, so that their ill health will not prevent them from pursuing that which is subjectively meaningful to them. The first possibility is not a convincing premise to explain the development of medicine. Species have survived and thrived for millennia without the benefit of physicians, even if others have not. Moreover, if one subscribes to the Darwinian notion of evolutionary pressure and survival of the fittest, the progress of medicine might even be seen as a regressive development, since medical interventions often accommodate the feeble and infirm, infringing on the process of natural selection. If some novel pathogen were to threaten the existence of humankind, it would likely be public health measures, rather than rescue of countless individual cases, that would protect the species.

The second possibility mentioned above, that the practice of medicine is primarily a societal endeavor born of utilitarian pragmatism, does have a cold, rational appeal but cannot account for many of the humanistic traditions that form the art. It is tempting to say that "the purpose" of medicine, assuming that there is only one or primarily one, is to ensure that individual citizens are healthy enough to contribute to the common good, and that their maladies and infirmities should not become a burden to society. This concept of medicine as a tool of societal efficiency, of which individual people are incidental beneficiaries, is more an ideological abstraction than a historical reality. While certain cultures and societies presumed that there were some people upon whom resources should not be wasted, and thus were forsaken in the name of Utopian efficiency, the societies themselves tended to perish along with their disprized citizens. It appears rather that it was those societies for which medicine was part of a more charitable and empathetic nature that thrived into modernity. It seems that a culture requires more than rational efficiency and cold calculation in order to prosper.

While medicine may be some part of human survival strategy or a utilitarian invention in support of communal efficiency, modern medicine is shaped primarily by the interactions of care-givers with individual patients, who receive care because of their individual circumstance rather than more general concerns.

The ancient Greeks did not conceive of Lachesis as a deity that measured the average lifespan of a population, or as concerned with the effects of plagues and epidemics on the course of history. The Fates were not actuaries, but rather made their determinations with great specificity for individual persons. The practitioners of the arts and science of medicine applied their skills with a similar focus. They treated and addressed themselves to the maladies of individual patients rather than homogenous communities. They undertook to relieve suffering of, restore health to, and forestall death in particular people.

Medicine had a different, more subjective focus than did the general health-promoting efforts of public health programs, and it is easy to surmise the reasons for this. For one, public health programs were most effective in averting certain communicable or infectious diseases. Diseases such as cancer, rheumatoid arthritis or epilepsy were not sufficiently sensitive to behavioral changes to benefit from a public health approach, particularly given the relative state of ignorance regarding their cause. Even today, when our understanding of the pathogenesis of cancer and heart disease is significantly more advanced, and public health efforts directed at education and healthful living are prevalent, these diseases affect a large portion of the population. It is highly unlikely that certain diseases such as hemophilia or Parkinson's Disease will yield to acceptable public health efforts that do not involve eugenics or other dystopian interventions.

There are reasons why one-on-one treatment of disease developed and the art and science of medicine advanced along with human understanding. As mentioned, humans tend to use tools when they are helpful to achieve a desired end, or avoid an undesirable one. Illness, injury, and disease cause suffering, and it is natural to apply the tools of human reason and observation to the plight of an afflicted individual. It would be expected that efforts would arise to improve the ordeal of childbirth, stabilize a broken limb, or ease the plight of consumptives. It may be less obvious why we would dialyze a demented octogenarian, or subject a child to the ordeal of multiple courses of progressively ineffective chemotherapy, but the principles underlying such efforts are probably not too different than those that motivated physicians in antiquity.

That physicians treat individual patients is not surprising; veterinarians treat individual animals and mechanics repair individual cars. Each of these remedial endeavors is rational from the perspective of efficiency and improving function when such interventions are expected to have sufficient long-term benefits. On the other hand, cars get junked and animals get put down, outcomes that modern medicine has not embraced, even when medical treatment objectively seems doomed to failure. There is an aspect to medical treatment of human beings that transcends utilitarian considerations. The development of this principle seems rational, even if its application in specific circumstances is not.

One of the reasons that modern medicine pours often heroic resources into the care of individual patients is the notion that the individuality of human beings makes them irreplaceable, and that whatever the state of life in the presence of disease or critical injury, each life might still possess some measure of meaningfulness to someone. It is these twin concepts of uniqueness and meaningfulness that endow modern medicine with perseverance past the point of diminishing, or even expected, returns. The reason why the farmer would be willing to replace, and euthanize his plow horse is because the horse is replaceable; philosophy and experience has convinced us that human beings are not. As many step-children may attest, it is not easy to substitute a parent, or easily transfer the affections that have developed as a grandparent enters her dotage. The ancients probably noticed that exceptional art was produced primarily by exceptional artists and that they could not be replaced by random conscription from the general public. Human beings are unique, and reason and sentiment lead us to suspect that such uniqueness is important.

We are also heirs of a thought tradition that believes that human life is meaningful, and that what is meaningful about an individual life is as specific as any other characteristic by which we can identify that person as unique. Thus, we conclude that it is not the province of the collective, or indeed anyone other than the affected person, to prescribe what is and is not meaningful in life, or whether a life is or is not worth living. It is possible that the most meaningful activity in a man's life after suffering a stroke is simply to hold his daughter's hand as she sits quietly at his bedside, waiting for the inevitable. It would be presumptuous to scoff at the octogenarian who wishes only to live long enough to see her granddaughter wed, or at the cancer patient whose life is meaningful as long as he can watch the dawn break. We as a civilization have consciously turned away from the notion that people, like pulleys and sprockets, have useful life spans and then wear out. We do not agree that when that utilitarian criterion is reached, there is no reason to opt for anything other than the most efficient form of disposal.

It is tempting to surmise that the idea that each individual life is unique, and thus entitled to pursue that which is subjectively meaningful, arises from religious dogma or romantic notions about the place of man in the universe. It is also possible to see how such a conclusion can be deduced from evidence that is readily observable. Our ancestors likely noticed that some people were smarter than others, that certain people were more pleasant to be around than were their colleagues, or that some were endowed with martial talents that were lacking in the rest. It is readily apparent, on the most cursory of examinations, that humans are unique and this uniqueness is not a trivial characteristic or one to be discarded lightly. We might expect that our ancestors, no less than ourselves, noticed that when a particular person died, something was lost forever.

Just as human beings can conclude that every life is special in some way, they can also infer from experience that life quite possibly has a point and that certain activities, experiences, and relations in life are meaningful. Such an inference is by no means mandatory, but it is at least understandable if we believe that there are reasons why people form emotional bonds with each other, develop and pursue ambitions, and derive both pleasure and satisfaction from various endeavors. If one considers these observations with the notion that many religious and philosophical traditions presume that life is, or can be, meaningful, it is natural to conclude that individual people live their lives in a way that seems meaningful to them. This conclusion gives medicine a focus beyond antagonism of the certainty of dying. The purpose of modern medicine might reasonably be supposed to be to limit the effect that disease and injury have on individual people's ability to live their lives in the way that is most meaningful to them.

Of course, it is a great oversimplification to assume that medicine, modern or otherwise, has a single purpose, or that such a purpose does not evolve over time. The principle that human beings are tool users applies to just about anything that humans can exploit for their own interests, including ancient and venerable institutions.

Medicine inherently subsumes the human qualities of compassion and charity. This fact can be observed by noting the histories of the many hospitals whose name begins with "Saint," "Presbyterian" or other denomination, as well as less overtly religious institutions such as the Shriner's hospitals. Medicine is naturally motivated by qualities such as empathy and human concern for the suffering of others. This does not mean, however, that when institutions have grown and thrived in the spirit of such noble motives they will not be exploited for profit, political advantage, or less altruistic personal interests. Medicine has a significant influence on culture and there is no reason to believe that the converse is not also true.

Healing is a prominent part of the social structure of many, if not all cultures. It would seem a logical attribute of survival instincts to be on the good side of someone thought to have the ability to cure illness, and relieve suffering. Likewise it would seem inevitable that such healers would occupy respected positions within the immediate community, as did the physicians of ancient Greece, Native American medicine men or the shamans of central Asia. Such respect was not merely a matter of protocol, as the ability to heal was naturally associated with other abilities of importance to the community. The shamans, for example, were believed to be intermediaries with the spiritual world, interceding there not only on behalf of the ill, but also for the tribe or community in general. Even in the absence of such mystical beliefs, healers would be looked upon as possessing a measure of wisdom that they acquire through their experiences of tending to the sick and dying. The healing arts, whatever their bases, allow their practitioners to observe the vulnerabilities of powerful people, the fears of the courageous, and the foolishness of the clever. Healers see life stripped of pretense and artifice and may acquire insights that are obscure to everyday experience.

Modern medicine is an amalgam of science and art, virtue and vice. It is a product of reason, emotion and mystical belief. It both influences and is influenced by the broader culture, and either directly or indirectly affects the life of nearly everyone on the planet. Modern medicine is an institution of triumphs and failures, of facts and myths. It is the latest stage in a metamorphosis that parallels civilization, and is sustained by the idea that human life is not an ordinary thing.

2

DISEASE

Disease is a common occurrence in human life, and human beings are naturally disposed to try and understand it. This has led people to devise various models of illness to allow them to analyze, explain and predict the course of their afflictions. Modeling is an essential part of human cognition, because if people could not construct models they would largely be unable to think. A thought, after all, is merely a model of whatever it is that one is thinking about.

The model that one adopts of a particular disease, or of disease in general, affects the approach to therapy, as well as the impact that diseases have on one's life. The diversity of models and theories of disease helps explain the emergence of various medical traditions, such as western and eastern approaches, as well as different therapeutic approaches within these broad traditions. Thus, for example, western medicine consists not only of conventional medicine and surgery, but also chiropractic, homeopathy, naturopathy, chelation therapy and prayer-based systems.

People adopt particular models of disease for various reasons. Some may choose a particular theory that is consistent with their general worldview. Others opt for concepts in which disease is largely preventable or curable if certain practices are followed and others avoided. Different people may be attracted to beliefs that give their particular maladies meaning within their own lives, or provide a framework that makes it easier to accept the disruptions that diseases sometimes cause.

Some people view disease as primarily a nutritional defect. They believe that their complaints and symptoms are caused by a deficiency of something that nature otherwise provides in the environment, and if that something would merely be incorporated into the diet, health would follow. Such people are convinced of the medicinal properties of herbs and extracts, and look to things like shark cartilage to treat cancer and garlic to manage high blood pressure. The fact that many plants and other naturally occurring substances have established medicinal effects provides at least some support for this approach.

Other people believe that diseases are largely the result of pathogens that enter their lives in one way or another. One subgroup of such people attribute their malaise or joint pains to environmental agents such as mold, or water impurities, or food additives. Others subscribe to a more fluid definition of what qualifies as a pathogen and include things like psychological stress, electromagnetic radiation, and atmospheric conditions. The widely accepted scientific principle that certain things do cause disease, like viruses, carcinogens and asbestos, permits supporters of this view to at least cite examples and reason by analogy.

Another concept of disease is that it is retribution for unwise lifestyle choices, or other lapses in living an ideal life. Ill health, in this view, is an expected consequence of indulgent behavior and unhealthful attitudes. Type 2 diabetes in obese patients, and smoking-related lung disease conform roughly to this descriptive model, but people who view their maladies in this way tend to do so more from a holistic and philosophical perspective. A similar model views disease as a matter of balance among environmental influences, psychological factors and salutary habits. Disease is thus a form of disharmony that can be remedied by some method of restoring the natural balance. Other people view physical illness as a manifestation of spiritual illness and, as in the case of Christian Science practitioners, seek cures through spiritual means.

The western medical tradition has been willing to adapt models and create new ones to accommodate reason, empirical observation and scientific investigation. While many people still prefer models of disease that deviate to varying degrees from a purely rationalist approach, most people accept that there is benefit to scientifically based medicine. When they are severely injured in an automobile accident or experience chest pain with difficulty breathing, most people do not direct paramedics to take them to organic gardeners or exorcists.

People, for the most part, trust science because science has a pretty good track record. Daily life presents ample evidence of the triumphs of science, from electronics to transportation to agriculture. Science and human reason have a pretty good resume and it is not surprising that progress in the diagnosis and treatment of disease and injury are almost exclusively made through advances in science. Because of abundant examples of the ability of science to make their lives better, people submit to science-based healthcare. They assume the benefit of computed tomography scans; they take pills, capsules and tablets that appear unremarkable but are reputed to have nearly magical effects on the human body; they submit to magnetic resonance imaging and minimally invasive procedures that can rearrange the configuration of some remote part of the body and require no more than a day or two of convalescence.

The scientific concept of disease is inextricably linked with the idea of modeling. The scientific approach utilizes several different models in identifying, classifying, studying, and analyzing disease states. Scientific investigation of a disease begins with identifying some process that affects people in an undesirable way, such as killing them, or making them feel miserable or unpleasant to be around. The most basic model is thus what may be termed a "descriptive model." Some astute individual makes an observation that a number of people begin to complain of similar symptoms, or demonstrate some behavior that varies noticeably from the accustomed norm. Hippocrates made detailed records of such observations in his *Epidemics*, and his ability to observe and describe pathologic processes is one reason why his favorable reputation in medicine persists to this day. The name "bubonic plague" derives from the buboes, or enlarged lymph nodes of the neck that occurred in patients afflicted with that disease, and thus the "black death" was understood initially as a description of its clinical effects. One modern example of such a descriptive model is that of the infection caused by the human immunodeficiency virus (HIV), and the consequent acquired immunodeficiency syndrome (AIDS). The disease entity was identified when an astute clinician noticed a number of homosexual men with the rare malignancy Kaposi sarcoma. His initial description of the phenomenon, though perhaps suspected of being caused by an infectious pathogen, was initially called "gay related immunodeficiency" or GRID. The earliest models of many diseases are simply descriptions of the observable effect that they have on patients or affected groups.

When our understanding of a disease or, more commonly, a symptom complex does not progress beyond this descriptive understanding patients and clinicians alike are invited to let their imaginations run wild with all sorts of causative associations and proposed therapies. This is frequently the case with symptom complexes such as chronic fatigue syndrome, fibromyalgia, or irritable bowel syndrome. While people who have been given one of these diagnoses no doubt suffer from something, the lack of more detailed models of their afflictions limits the ability of cold, objective science to provide them relief.

Another type of model that is useful in the scientific practice of medicine is an association model. This type of model aggregates certain objective data about a given disease, without requiring understanding of why a particular datum is important. These data are then used to help derive some understanding of, and allow predictions about, where diseases occur. Certain diseases, like atherosclerotic heart disease are linked with identified risk factors, such as diabetes, high blood pressure, cigarette smoking, and family history. Even if nothing more were known about coronary artery disease, these associations would allow clinicians to describe populations at risk for heart attack and stroke. Early in the history of the AIDS epidemic researchers noticed a correlation between infection with the human immunodeficiency virus and certain types of hepatitis. This allowed at least a crude method of screening for possible HIV infection to try and identify infected patients before the telltale collapse of the body's immune system. Efforts to combat malaria by controlling mosquitoes and religious dietary laws that had the effect of mitigating food-borne illness may also have been the products of such modeling.

A more detailed model that results from scientific inquiry is what might be termed a causation model. This not only notices an association between two observations related to a particular disease, but also identifies a causal connection between the two. The identification of certain chemicals in cigarette smoke as causative agents in lung cancer, or the identification of the human immunodeficiency virus as the pathogen responsible for AIDS are examples of causation models. Laboratory investigations can establish the relationship between some disease process and a suspected cause. This is an intermediate step on the road to the scientific understanding of the pathogenesis and mechanism of the disease being considered.

Even if a causal link between a disease process and some external phenomenon is established, the exact mechanism responsible for the disease condition may remain obscure. This was true when the human immunodeficiency virus was first identified, but the exact mechanism by which it attacked the immune system was unknown.

The ultimate goal of the scientific modeling of disease is the pathophysiologic model, a detailed description of the precise mechanisms by which disease occurs in the body. Such models describe, for example, the role of particular genes in the development of cancerous tumors, and how the age related decline in certain hormones leads to osteoporosis. Intensive study of HIV led to intricate knowledge of how the virus was transmitted, invaded and corrupted the immune system and led to the demise of those infected with it. Knowledge of the complex processes in the virus's replication, interaction with the host and survival mechanisms allowed the development of rational and elegant therapies, with the eventual goal of eradication of the pathogen from an infected patient. One goal of medical science is to develop as detailed understandings as possible of the diseases that afflict humans. This allows rational development of accurate diagnostic methods and effective prevention and treatment strategies.

The pathophysiologic model is the goal of scientific investigation regarding disease, since its aim is a complete understanding of the risk factors, cause, course, effects on the body and outcome of particular diseases. These are items that naturally curious human minds will seek to understand and predict, consistent with our desire to investigate and understand life's circumstances in general. In the absence of scientifically developed and verified understanding of disease processes, people tend to do what they do regarding other important areas where they lack sufficient information: they fill in the blanks by using surrogates for the missing knowledge. These surrogates include analogies, personification, superstition or guessing. As is the case with the descriptive models described above, if all that people are presented with are observed associations or causal links, they are free to propose all manner of prevention strategies, mechanisms responsible for sickness, and candidate therapies. Probably the most familiar example of an association between a phenomenon and an illness, one that nonetheless lacks a causal link or established mechanism, is the perception that the common cold is caused by cold weather. Other examples can be found in the medical media, which occasionally publish studies linking, for example, high voltage power lines with childhood leukemia, cell phone use with brain tumors, vaccines with autism, and residence at higher latitudes with multiple sclerosis. Many lifestyle habits or consumer goods are preliminarily linked to some malady, with the association disappearing on closer scrutiny. The first few years of AIDS therapy created a correlation between those taking HIV medicines and those suffering AIDS symptoms, causing at least some people to conclude that the medicines used to treat HIV infection caused AIDS.

Many diseases are now so well understood that medical science has developed highly accurate diagnostic methods and therapies that, even if they do not cure those diseases, allow them to be managed so as to have as little impact as possible on the affected person's life. Examples of such diseases include many types of cancer, rheumatoid arthritis, diabetes and gout. Even though medical science has supposedly provided complete models and effective therapy, however, many people still adhere to other models of disease for various reasons. They still believe that shark cartilage or antioxidants cure cancer, or that patients can only truly be freed from a given disease by prayer.

People have a variety of motivations for believing certain things about their health, and maintain those beliefs even when doing so seems objectively self-defeating. The situation is particularly obvious the less that is known about what causes a particular disease, or what treatment works best, or even whether or not something can be considered a disease. If, for example, there is some doubt as to which remedy works best for a particular condition, people are free to propose therapies, and their interest in proposing those therapies may not be the same as those of the patients seeking them. Modern medicine consists of many discrete, often competing, interests that do not agree on what constitutes a desirable outcome. Uncertainties that exist regarding what causes certain diseases, who gets them, how they are diagnosed, and how they might be treated create opportunities for the altruistic and the self-interested, the gifted healers and the quacks, the compassionate and the predators alike.

Diseases and illness affect nearly everyone's life at one time or another and therefore those people will have to contend with the accompanying uncertainties. It may be that people still prefer shark cartilage or prayer, not because they are ignorant about the biologic facts of disease but rather they are uncertain about what it means to them and how it affects larger questions in their lives.

Uncertainties abound in medicine, and this is not simply a result of ignorance or faulty investigation. There are some issues that have no satisfactory, universal resolution. For example, the two statements "why do people get sick?" and "what causes disease?" may be considered identical in one sense, but may also be viewed as unrelated queries, philosophical in the former case, scientific in the latter. The entire concept of cause is itself too indefinite to serve as a fixed star by which to navigate uncertainty. Aristotle recognized four different types of cause: material, formal, efficient and final. For example, the material cause of an automobile is the metal and plastic from which it is constructed. The formal cause is the design by which the car is built, the efficient cause is the workmen assembling the car in a factory and the final cause is the need of someone somewhere for transportation. A similar perspective-dependency afflicts questions of cause in medicine. If a diabetic person loses a foot to a non-healing infection, it might be said with equal validity that the person lost the foot because of inadequate treatment of his diabetes; because of the genetic and other factors related to developing diabetes; because of an unfortunate infection or vascular disease; or because of, quite simply, a surgeon who removed the foot with a saw.

The concept of uncertainty affects all facets of disease and, indeed, all facets of medicine. For a given disease in a given patient there may be uncertainty as to the diagnosis, the prognosis and expected course, the best treatment, the risk associated with various therapies, etc. There may even be uncertainty as to whether a person has a disease. If a grandmother forgets to mail her utility bill, does she have a disease? Does the weekend gardener who is increasingly bothered by the lingering aches that accompany her hobby have fibromyalgia, or the spirited second grader, attention deficit hyperactivity disorder? Many people take antidepressants, and it is at least worth wondering about the certainty of the diagnoses that justify the prescriptions. A casual observer might conclude that the number of people afflicted with a particular disease or set of symptoms increases when there is publicity regarding a new treatment for that condition.

Most anyone suffering a particular type of bothersome symptom seeks an explanation and understanding of the processes causing it. Knowledge can sometimes be comforting even if it is wrong, or based on faulty data. When medicine recognizes syndromes such as irritable bowel syndrome, or myofascial pain syndrome, or any other condition that does not have a single, defined cause, it becomes quite easy for physicians and other practitioners to bestow that diagnosis in a catch-all attempt to relieve some of the uncertainty that may be troubling a particular patient. For many people, a diagnosis, even if only a formal name that includes no information that the patient could not have figured out on his own, is a form of reassurance, and in its own way, a form of therapy. Thus, practitioners will often shoe-horn a set of confounding patient complaints into the definition of some poorly characterized disease state, tweaking the defining criteria as needed and expanding the population whose diseases have yet to be discovered.

One of the respected references of modern medical practice, *Dorland's Medical Dictionary*, defines disease as:

> any deviation from or interruption of the normal structure or function of any body part, organ, or system that is manifested by a characteristic set of symptoms and signs and whose etiology, pathology and prognosis may be known or unknown.

It should be instructive that this definition concedes that uncertainty regarding etiology, pathology, and prognosis, is an accepted phenomenon in describing and dealing with human disease. It is equally instructive to note that the etymology of the word disease is rather straightforward: It is from the Old French "des", meaning "without," and "aise," meaning comfort or contentment. The derivation of the word itself comes from subjective considerations rather than biological or pathological ones, and suggests that the practical effect of diseases is not so much on objective measures of health as on the subjective effect on the lives of those who suffer them.

One consequence of identifying diseases by clinical signs and subjective symptoms is that these do not always result from some derangement in the body's function. Symptoms in particular can result from psychological factors, or transient environmental influences. While these need not always indicate disease in the objective sense, they do frequently lead to diagnostic investigations and application of various therapies. Since the defining symptoms need not always result from some objective derangement in the body's structure or metabolic regulation, it is quite possible to have effective interventions other than those that are confirmed by medical science to counter the underlying mischief.

The practical effect of considering disease from the perspective of subjective symptoms and nonspecific signs is that it gives rise to a general definition that helps identify the benefits of the various types of healing arts: disease is any condition or perceived condition for which people seek intervention. The intervention may be self-medicating with any variety of agents, or seeking the skill of a practitioner, whether it is a physician, folk healer, shaman, naturopath, Christian Science practitioner, etc. It may be more satisfying, and more common to regard disease as an objective, potentially identifiable defect in the structure or function of the body, but the reality is that modern medicine, whatever the school or discipline, ultimately treats people when they do not feel right, regardless of the cause.

The term "disease" does not refer to a finite set of conditions that medical science is relentlessly trying to run down. Progress brings with it new maladies and new medical challenges. There is an entire set of conditions that become apparent only when other medical successes make longevity the norm. Alzheimer's disease is one such condition. Other diseases did not exist, or were at least unknown until modern methods of diagnosis and therapy were implicated in causing them. One such example is nephrogenic systemic fibrosis (NSF), a condition that occurs in dialysis patients who receive contrast agents for magnetic resonance imaging. As dialysis and magnetic resonance imaging were inventions of the twentieth century, NSF was unknown before that time. Even if medicine does not introduce completely new diseases it can alter the epidemiology and prevalence of older ones. This is likely the case with the diarrhea caused by the bacterium *clostridium difficile*. It is possible that the organism is ancient, but the clinically significant infection became widespread with the introduction of broad-spectrum antibiotics. Successful medical interventions do not always leave the body in the desired state.

Human progress has resulted in unintended medical issues, such as the diseases associated with obesity, a condition promoted by affluence and material progress. Other conditions, such as silicosis, and repetitive motion injuries are the result of industrialization, and there is in fact a discrete medical discipline devoted to occupational medicine.

The perception of disease does not always originate from disordered biology. Modern society has allowed for the "medicalizing" of behaviors that were once thought to be due to undesirable character traits. This is particularly apparent in psychology and psychiatry where many types of undesirable behaviors and difficulties are attributed to newly described disorders. These include sex and internet addiction, moodiness, public displays of anger, social phobias, stress, and substance abuse. Disagreeable people are suspected of having a personality disorder, or perhaps an undefined "chemical imbalance." One of the consequences of associating disease with the concepts of normal and abnormal is that it invites labeling as diseases not only those conditions that are objectively unhealthy, but also those that are undesirable or socially and culturally disfavored. While a purist may be tempted to scoff at labeling these behaviors as medical disorders, they do share with more conventional diseases the effect of interfering with some part of life that is important to the sufferer. Whether medical science, or other forms of healthcare have anything useful to offer in such circumstances is a matter that will only be resolved with experience.

It is difficult to have a comprehensive understanding of disease because of the varying effect that a given disease may have on different people, and because of the vast array of diseases that can affect the body. Even more generalized contemplation of disease in human life presents a paradox. Every human that has ever lived has had an experience of disease, either as the person afflicted or because of encounters with family or acquaintances who were. Experience with disease is normal in human life, yet disease is regarded as an abnormal state.

Despite the fact that the modern concept of diseases is somewhat inexact, the term "modern medicine" is generally understood to mean the scientifically-based discipline concerned with investigating, diagnosing and treating observable derangements in the body's structure or function. Human reason and the scientific method have been remarkably successful in this endeavor, and this success has followed from the realization that diseases arise in myriad ways, not always avoidable or treatable, and not arising from a single principle. If there is any underlying "cause" of disease, in the sense that Aristotle referred to a final cause, it is the complexity of the human organism.

The fact that diseases are so marked by uncertainty is a natural consequence of the fact that the human body and human activities are unfathomably complex. Everyday experience makes it easy for us to take for granted how truly remarkable the human body is. Even the simplest activities require the coordination and precise functioning of multiple systems. The very common act of getting out of bed involves moving from a posture where the heart and brain are approximately the same height, to one where the head is a foot or more above the level of the heart, and gravity tends to pull blood toward the now much lower feet. In the absence of a prompt and precise response to this change of circumstance, the blood pressure in the brain would rapidly fall and rising from bed would be reliably accompanied by collapsing on the floor. Likewise, when we consider the many conditions in which in which it is necessary for blood to circulate, it is amazing that it does not more commonly clot throughout our veins while sitting on the couch, or run out our ears when we sneeze. Even in the most ordinary circumstances, the typical human body is capable of, among other things, seeing, thinking, hearing, eating, smelling, ambulating, talking, feeling, planning, reproducing, growing, healing, throwing, balancing, grasping, and tasting. This list even understates the body's capabilities, since not only can the typical person see, he can pick out a face in a crowd; not only can he hear, he can localize the direction from which a sound originates; he can not only walk, but do so at a range of different speeds; he can not only grasp an object, but also manipulate it so as to assume any desired orientation with respect to the body.

Yet another degree of complexity results from the body's ability to adapt to different conditions. The amount of blood that the heart pumps per minute can increase approximately five fold as the body goes from a state of rest to one of strenuous exercise. The body can avidly retain fluid when intake is restricted and expel large excess volumes when necessary to avoid overload. Similarly, humans can live in temperature extremes of about 140 degrees Fahrenheit while regulating their body temperature to within one or two degrees for short periods of time. The capacity to adapt includes the ability to repair injuries and fight off invading pathogens such as viruses and bacteria, to build muscle in response to weight-bearing activity and to store excess nutrients for later use. The necessity of adapting requires the capacity to change, and the changes are not always in the direction of better health.

All of the sophisticated processes, complex functions, and capacity to adapt can give rise to diseases. The failure to adapt sufficiently to some environmental change might be regarded as abnormal, as can an inappropriate attempt to adapt when there is no stimulus to do so. It is easy to imagine that the processes by which the body produces new tissue in response to injury or physical exertion might become disordered and produce cancerous growths, or that the process by which the body's immune system adapts to confront countless potential pathogens might, through very small imperfections, become directed at the body's own structures and produce conditions such as lupus and rheumatoid arthritis. It is similarly easy to appreciate how some small imperfection in the body's ability to adapt to different environments might make it susceptible to illness from a novel microbe. These small vulnerabilities in the body's defenses are in fact a necessary consequence of the ability to adapt at all. Nature has chosen sexual reproduction as the strategy for ensuring genetic diversity and the survival advantage that it provides for the species. Different people will have different genetic traits, and thus different responses to external conditions. In order for the species to survive in a wide variety of environments, it is unavoidable that different people will vary in their ability to adapt to a given condition. Some will be more accommodating of environmental perturbations than others, and it is a statistical certainty that there will be some who will not be accommodating at all.

An accessible model of disease is suggested by Stephen Hawking's example of entropy given in his book *A Brief History of Time*. Dr. Hawking described a billiards table and noted that the position of the balls just after being racked is only one of an innumerable set of possible positions, and that it is highly unlikely that, once this initial position is disturbed, a single shot would return all of the balls to it. In a similar fashion, all of the body's processes, functions and structures might have a configuration of perfect health, analogous to the well-ordered billiard balls after racking, but given the complexity of the organism, the multitude of ways that things can go wrong, and the challenges that it faces, it is unlikely that such a state of ordered health will be maintained.

Disease is an ever-changing entity. It is likely to be with us, in constantly changing forms as long as we are here. New diseases arise from myriad sources, including the cures for older ones, and old diseases are found to have been nothing more normal variations, or different manifestations of something more familiar. Despite the natural association of disease with the abnormal, the one characteristic of disease that is unlikely to ever change is that it is common.

3

DIAGNOSIS

Human beings have an aversion to the unknown. It is contrary to the natural human trait of curiosity to leave matters of practical importance unexamined. People want to know about the conditions that cause them distress, impair their abilities or shorten their lives. They want to know what is wrong with them, what to do about it and what the outcome is likely to be. For these reasons, as well as the practical reality that a correct identification of the malady is sometimes crucial to proper treatment, diagnosis is an inherent part of the practice of modern medicine.

The search for a diagnosis is often a prerequisite to appropriate therapy, but the process is also one that shapes the therapeutic relationship. It seems intuitive that patients would have an unalterable interest in reaching an accurate diagnosis, but in practice this is not always the case. Patients are sometimes not accepting of irrefutable evidence of a given diagnosis when one is presented and are similarly reluctant to assist the practitioner in arriving at those diagnoses. Some patients harbor latent superstitions regarding the obscure institutions of modern medicine and will not abandon their views in submission to what they regard as technologically advanced alchemy. It is sometimes the case that a patient will suspect that his symptoms are the result of some grave untreatable condition, and will not relay his suspicions to his physician, or even admit to consistent symptoms. This behavior apparently arises from the theory that if he has the condition, modern medicine will find it without his help, but if his fears are unfounded he does not want to lead the investigation to conclusions that he would rather avoid.

Not all diagnoses have the same implications, and the same diagnosis has different implications for different people. Huntington's disease, for example, is a uniformly debilitating genetic condition, and there are tests to identify those persons whose lives will be affected by it. Some people would want to know this, others would not.

Besides the implications of a particular diagnosis for a patient, the process of diagnosis is central to the value of medicine as a human institution. While a given diagnosis might be devastating news for one patient, it might provide comfort and reassurance to another. One patient may regard a diagnosis of lung cancer as a pronouncement that his life is now out of his control, while the same information may lead another patient to conclude that he now has the information needed to plan the remainder of his life in manner most meaningful to him.

The physician-patient relationship is often validated by the ability of the practitioner to provide a diagnosis, even if it eventually turns out to be wrong, or otherwise unhelpful. Diagnoses are often points of reference for patients in incorporating physical signs and symptoms into their daily lives, and can determine whether the patient and practitioner will maintain a beneficial relationship.

The essence of diagnosis is the collection of various pieces of information about a patient's complaints and then drawing inferences from those pieces to reach a conclusion as to the patient's condition. The word comes directly from the Greek, meaning "a discerning or distinguishing." It is an intensely cognitive endeavor that involves more than mechanical application of rigid rules to clinical data. Despite the ideal that a diagnosis be an objectively provable fact, arrived at logically, and precisely determined by reliable and specific data, the actual process of reaching a diagnosis remains as much an art as a science.

The process of diagnosis often attempts to characterize extremely complex and often poorly understood processes by examining a relatively sparse collection of clues. Sometimes the available data are sufficient for the task. Finding an abnormally high level of heart enzymes in the blood is reliably associated with heart attack for example, although for a particular patient other information is necessary to provide definitive treatment, such as determining the location of the damage, and assessing the function of the heart in the setting of such damage. Certain therapies, such as giving an aspirin or blood thinners, do not require these more detailed data, but more definitive care, such as angioplasty or heart bypass surgery, usually requires more than a general confirmation that the heart has been damaged. The process of diagnosis is often an ongoing endeavor seeking more specific and detailed information upon which to base clinical decisions.

The raw materials of diagnosis are clinical data related to the patient's condition. These data consist initially of the patient's symptoms and externally observable signs of disease. These are then supplemented by various clues that might be found by inquiring into the patient's past history, family history and habits. Further data may come from a variety of sources, such as clinical laboratory studies, radiographs or other medical images of the body, epidemiologic data, and descriptions of other patient's with similar complaints. Ideally, these data are used to first develop a list of potential diagnoses, and then narrow that list as additional information is obtained. This process works very well in the abstract, as well as for those conditions with distinctive and exclusive clinical characteristics. It dramatically understates the skill and experience needed to make accurate diagnoses in many of the most common conditions, however.

The difficulties begin with the patient's complaints of symptoms. These are often vague and non-specific, such as pain, dizziness or nausea. Many complaints, such as abdominal pain have dozens of potential causes, and the patient is often unable to convey sufficient additional information to narrow the possibilities. Most symptoms, by themselves, do not contain enough information to conclusively identify a cause, even with reliable and thorough descriptions of the distressing phenomena and their accompanying sensations. The situation is similar to that in which someone proposes to describe an animal to you and ask you to guess what it is. The description may be something like "the animal is brown, four legged, has fur or hair, a tail and a long neck." There is significant data there, but none of it provides enough detail to arrive at a specific answer. Is it a dog, a horse, a deer, or something more exotic? The information given may allow deductions regarding potentially useful information, such as that the animal is a vertebrate, warm-blooded and reproduces sexually, but these are still characteristics that provide no help in answering the specific question posed. Similar situations commonly arise in medicine, when patients seek information about some symptom complex, and the available data may allow little more than an educated guess as to the diagnosis.

Missing or incomplete data is a common reality in modern medicine. Information necessary to make a conclusive diagnosis is frequently absent, inaccessible or inconsistent. Sometimes information that, in retrospect, seems to make the process of diagnosis trivial was not available or not appreciated in the midst of a patient's crisis. Medical practitioners usually do not have the advantages of a car mechanic; they cannot take their patients apart, examine the pieces and put them back together again, nor can they swap out parts and see if that fixes the problem. Even if theoretically accessible, some clinical information may not provide sufficient benefit to justify the expense, risk and physical burden on the patient that is involved with collecting it. Some syndromes may not have specific findings that conclusively determine their presence or absence; for example there is no reliable laboratory assay that confirms the presence of, or distinguishes different causes of pain.

Clinicians who are faced with these gaps in diagnostic information resort to the same compensatory practices used when there is missing information about diseases, or indeed to accommodate incomplete information in virtually any area of human experience: collecting surrogate data, drawing inferences from known data or patterns in data, making assumptions, and taking educated guesses that may be influenced by experience, emotion or ancillary considerations.

The use of surrogate information is very common in medicine. One example is the measurement of serum creatinine to evaluate kidney function. It is frequently necessary for physicians to know if the kidneys are filtering blood normally. In determining this they need to know how much blood is being filtered by the kidneys, as opposed to just flowing through them on the way back to the heart. Direct measurement of this quantity is challenging and impractical for most clinical purposes. Physicians thus identified a molecule in the blood that, to a reasonable approximation, is almost completely filtered by the kidney, and is readily measured in both the blood and the urine. These two values can then be compared and the amount of blood cleared of creatinine calculated. Reasonable assumptions can then be used to estimate the rate at which the kidney filters blood, and this can be used to determine how well the kidney performs this task in a given patient at a given time. Experience has led physicians to cut out many of the intermediate calculations, however, and it frequently happens that kidney function is estimated not from calculation of the filtration rate of the kidney, but by simple measurement of the blood creatinine. Thus, the difficulty of obtaining a particular clinical parameter, i.e. the rate at which the kidney filters blood, is accommodated by use of a clinically convenient surrogate, measurement of blood creatinine.

Upon close inspection, many common clinical data are found to be surrogates for less accessible information. The common chest x-ray is used frequently to evaluate for pneumonia, fluid in the lungs, heart enlargement, collapsed lung, rib fractures, etc., but in reality an x-ray is simply a two dimensional map of the relative transparency of chest structures to radiation of certain frequencies. Cutting edge technologies such as positron emission tomography (PET scanning) and enzyme linked immunosorbent-assays (ELISA) directly measure quantities that are surrogates for the diagnostic information of interest. The common pulse oximeter does not directly measure blood oxygen saturation;

it measures the relative intensity of reflected light at different frequencies and uses this information to derive an estimate of how much oxygen is in the blood. Likewise, the electrocardiogram that is a staple of cardiac diagnosis is simply a graphical representation of bioelectric signals measured on the surface of the chest. Surrogate data, not being perfectly correlated with the information of interest, may be affected by phenomena other than those representing the desired data. A hazy shadow on a chest x-ray may represent pneumonia, a scar from a previous pathologic process, a tumor, hemorrhage, or other abnormality. The quantity being measured, the two-dimensional distribution of radiation transparencies, may be similar in each of these cases, requiring some degree of interpretation or consideration of other data in arriving at the correct diagnosis.

Despite a degree of uncertainty that accompanies the use of surrogate data, it is usually not necessary for such data to correlate perfectly with the clinical parameter of interest; indeed such inerrant correlation almost never exists. The kidney adds creatinine to urine by processes other than filtration; thus, while measurement of creatinine gives a clinically useful estimate of the filtering function of a patient's kidneys, it is not 100% accurate. Shadows on x-rays are caused by phenomena other than pneumonia, and pulse oximeter readings are influenced by factors other than the oxygen content of the patient's blood. All of these examples illustrate that using surrogate data creates a potential source of error in collecting accurate information about a patient's diagnosis.

When collection of surrogate data is either insufficient or not possible, diagnosticians must resort to other strategies to make up for missing, incomplete or conflicting clinical data. Experienced clinicians often draw inferences from known data or characteristic patterns in the data. One example is when physicians inquire into a family history of disease or consider similarity in symptoms in order to narrow potential diagnoses and plan therapeutic interventions. Other examples might be analysis of blood samples to determine red blood cell size or the presence of enzymes produced by the liver to evaluate for the presence of heavy alcohol use. Heart muscle damage is seldom directly observed, and its presence is almost always inferred from finding abnormal levels of certain heart related enzymes circulating in the blood. Hepatitis is diagnosed by discovering inflammation in the liver, along with identifying certain antibodies or other chemical evidence of a causative pathogen, but its presence may be suspected by observing a yellowish tint to the patients eyes or reports that the patient's urine has turned dark brown. These findings are suggestive of jaundice and are related to the build up of bilirubin, a waste product that results from the natural life cycle of red blood cells. As is the case with surrogate data however, the inferences drawn from clinical data are often non-specific, and although they may be suggestive of certain diagnoses, they are not conclusive. Jaundice, for example can also result from blockage of the bile duct by gallstones, or an abnormal destruction of red blood cells by certain disease processes. Dark urine may also result from certain medications, metabolic diseases unrelated to liver inflammation, or the abnormal breakdown of skeletal muscle.

Because surrogate data, and the data used to produce inferences are usually nonspecific, these data must be interpreted to provide clinically useful information. Radiologists spend five years in residency honing their ability to provide interpretations of imaging studies. Likewise cardiologists, kidney specialists, psychiatrists, surgeons, and every other clinician that undertakes to treat illness and injury spend years learning the subtle art of interpreting the clinical clues relevant to their areas of practice.

Interpretations of data are also data. It is routine for a clinician to consider a radiologist's interpretation of an x-ray in the process of diagnosis, or to incorporate his or her own interpretation of laboratory data in sorting out the source of a patient's complaint. Even data that would seem to definitively reveal or rule out a particular condition require interpretation. Cultures of blood to search for evidence of bacterial infection may grow such bacteria when they are present in the blood, but also when they have inadvertently been inoculated into the culture medium during the collection process. In such cases, the results must be interpreted in the setting of other clinical data in order to avoid erroneous conclusions.

The reliance of medical diagnosis on interpretations of data has several implications for modern medicine. The additional step of interpretation creates an opportunity for error to enter into the process, and even the most meticulous diagnostic work up and data collection can be vitiated by errors in interpretation. Furthermore, interpretation of data inevitably results in the loss of detail otherwise contained within those data. There is a reason why a review of a two and a half hour movie takes only three minutes to read. The situation is the same with interpretations of electrocardiogram tracings, x-ray results, or laboratory data. It is often desirable for the data interpreter to get to the bottom line and declare an EKG to be "normal" or a radiologist to identify an infiltrate on chest x-ray that is consistent with pneumonia. This is often an efficient method of presenting complex information to the clinician in a form useful to the task of diagnosis, but such interpretations often omit subtle details present in the raw data. For example, the identification of an infiltrate on a chest radiograph, by itself, does not provide information that distinguishes different causes of infiltrates. The omitted details may not be especially relevant to the immediate interpretation of the study in question, but such detail may be quite useful in the primary effort of determining a diagnosis.

Diagnostic processes that rely heavily on the interpretation of various data are subject to another source of inaccuracy, and that derives from the cognitive influences that affect interpretation. Pattern recognition is an inherent part of human data processing, and requires a certain amount of flexibility in recognizing associations between diagnostic data and diagnostic conclusions. Apophenia is the psychological phenomenon by which a person perceives a pattern in what is otherwise random data, such as when someone identifies a face in a rust stain, or sees animal shapes in clouds. Apophenia can have a powerful influence on what conclusions are drawn from clinical data, and in the realm of medical diagnosis this tendency can be exacerbated by the large amounts of data supplied by modern medical technology. There may be a tendency to jump to conclusions on sketchy data, or to abandon a correct diagnosis when some of the data do not seem to fit.

These pitfalls are inherent in human reasoning and it is simply the reality that the process of making inferences involves a risk that those inferences may be wrong. It is certainly useful that we are able to pick out familiar faces in a crowd, and this capacity is made no less useful by the occasional experience when we mistake one person for another.

Apophenia is not abnormal; to the contrary it is a necessary consequence of the process of interpretation. This is so because of a paradox that arises when considering random data. This paradox is illustrated by considering a computer screen or television monitor. A random pattern would produce an image that is commonly referred to as "snow," the visual equivalent of white noise. This results from a random distribution of picture elements of different shades or colors. If we were to divide the screen up into a certain number of squares, say 100, we can then quantify the number of picture elements of a given shade or color in each. If it happened that one square contained three times the average number of elements of a particular shade than any other square, it would seem natural to ask what caused the concentration. It would appear that the abnormally high concentration represents a pattern produced by some cause. It would be expected that randomness would result in approximately equal distributions of elements in all 100 squares, yet, if each square had exactly the same number of elements of each shade or color, this distribution would in fact represent not randomness but a describable and predictable pattern. For human cognition to be useful to human activity, the mind must be capable of perceiving patterns in data or configurations that are both the result of specific causes, or that might result from simple random variation and coincidence.

The quality of data upon which healthcare practitioners rely to make medical diagnoses is affected not only by technical considerations, but also the interaction between patient and practitioner. Patients are not always forthcoming with, or truthful about relevant clinical information, such as alcohol or drug use, or the frequency of symptoms. Some patients seek medical care for reasons other than improving or maintaining their health, such as to obtain narcotics, procure medical excuses legitimizing lack of ambition or success in outside endeavors, or to medicalize stresses that are otherwise unrelated to their physical health. All of these influences affect the process of medical diagnosis and occasionally lead to diagnostic inaccuracy. Technology can help minimize the tendency to error but not eliminate it, and medical diagnosis will remain something of an art for the foreseeable future. Most medical tests have associated with them performance statistics describing how good they are at detecting a condition when it is present, and not detecting it when it is not. For most modern medical applications, the errors associated with clinical data are minor or can be accommodated by other means. The fact that they are there, however, should counsel caution that, even in the setting of dazzling technological advances, modern diagnosis is not infallible.

When diagnostic data are missing, inaccurate or misinterpreted, the result is often an incorrect diagnosis. Wrong diagnoses are an inherent part of medicine and can have a variety of consequences. Diagnostic errors and omissions can lead to inappropriate, ineffective and potentially harmful therapies, and cause both unnecessary mental distress and false senses of relief. They can lead to the phenomenon of miracle cures when a condition is identified as some incurable malady, which then mysteriously improves on its own. Incorrect diagnoses are common in modern medicine, not due to incompetence or carelessness on the part of practitioners, but because of the enormous variety, variability and inconsistency of human diseases.

It may happen that a physician is asked to diagnose a condition that is yet unknown to modern medicine, or which has a unique presentation in a particular patient. Sometimes a patient is given a diagnosis of a particular condition because the practitioner cannot think of anything else to explain the symptoms. Other diagnoses are termed "diagnoses of exclusion," essentially defaults when there are no confirming data upon which to reach a more definite conclusion.

When modern physicians are in training, a prevailing notion is that the good doctor is the one who correctly makes an obscure diagnosis, or who arrives at correct diagnosis on the most subtle and sparse clinical data. This leads to the common practice of constructing differential diagnoses, i.e. lists of potential disease states, and then ordering laboratory and imaging studies suggested by each item on the list. It is common for physicians in training to equate the ordering of diagnostic tests with the practice of medicine. Such endeavors are often unrevealing, because the actual diagnosis may be hidden by atypical presentations, misleading test results and pertinent clinical clues that evade the physician's notice. Experience eventually leads to the reality that the truly gifted healer is the one who not only makes an appropriate diagnosis when possible, but who resists the temptation to pronounce a diagnosis just for the sake of having one. The skilled practitioner of the healing art is the one who is able to make the patient better, even if reasonable effort has not revealed the identity of the malady.

Diagnosis is an essential part of the practice of medicine, although it is one that is often inexact and frequently frustrating. Occasionally physicians will confront the temptation to proclaim a particular diagnosis because the patient expects one and they are otherwise stumped. Making and giving a patient a diagnosis is more than a prelude to either providing appropriate therapy, or concluding that therapy would be of no benefit. When a patient is told that he or she has a particular condition, the implications go beyond clinical management. Associating a particular disease with a patient may affect self-image, long-term goals and ambitions and approach to the remainder of life. It is one thing for a clinician to be "pretty sure" about the presence of disease based on a few clues, and quite another to relay the result of this accomplishment to a patient who may be devastated by the news. This is particularly significant when the disease in question is a degenerative one such as Parkinson's disease, or a terminal one such as metastatic cancer. In some settings the pressure on the clinician to make a diagnosis is greater than that to be accurate, because the clinician perceives that the uncertainty is unduly distressing.

Patients sometimes refuse to accept that the cause of their complaints and ailments has escaped discovery and thus end up with an unhelpful diagnosis of some ill-defined syndrome. Patients place a great deal of importance on diagnoses because a diagnosis implies various degrees of knowledge or certainty about the disease, such as what causes it, what course it will take and what to do about it. Some people are just happy that their condition has a name, implying that other people have it too, and validating their symptoms. Having a diagnosis makes the medical adversary less mysterious and thus less menacing. Sometimes merely having a diagnosis is therapeutic, even if the diagnosis is wrong. Medical diagnosis is an art, if for no other reason than that it involves much more than simply identifying disease.

4

THERAPY

Once the practitioner arrives at a diagnosis of the patient's condition, an obvious question becomes "What is to be done about it?" As the medieval physician Paracelsus (1493-1541) reasonably wondered: "What sense would it make or what would it benefit a physician if he discovered the origin of the diseases but he could not cure or alleviate them?" The search for effective interventions to relieve the discomfort, disability and mortality of disease and trauma largely describes the history of medicine, and the effectiveness of those interventions determines the validity of the various concepts of healthcare.

Whether a particular intervention survives as an effective form of treatment for a disease or injury depends on the observed effectiveness of that intervention in practice. How a particular intervention came to be used as therapy depends largely on how people viewed the condition for which it was used. If the disease was perceived as a nutritional deficiency, dietary supplements would be a rational approach to treatment. Some conditions are caused by the lack of essential nutrients and replacement of the deficient substance is rational and effective therapy. Treatment of beriberi with thiamine and scurvy with vitamin C are obvious examples of this concept. As with many medical treatments, their effectiveness can be observed and incorporated into medical practice even though the precise mechanism by which they work is unknown. A Scottish surgeon, James Lind, discovered in 1753 that consumption of citrus fruits could cure scurvy, even though it was not until 1932 that vitamin C was identified as the deficient nutrient. It is highly unlikely that the Alpine shepherd whose frozen remains were found 5300 years after his death had any idea why the birch fungus he carried had medicinal benefits.

It seems reasonable to assume that certain forms of therapy arise because they make intuitive sense, such as bandaging a wound, or invoking divine intervention in cases where the patient believes that illness is the result of some spiritual concern. Acupuncture makes sense in the context of energy flows and meridians, even if the process seems occult to anyone who does not accept the underlying premises. Some substances just seem like they might make someone feel better, like the sap of the aloe vera plant. History does not retain the details of how the Quechua Indians of Peru came to recognize the therapeutic benefits of chincona bark and the quinine that it contained to reduce shivering in cold temperatures. Observation of its effects, however, led to hypotheses and trials that demonstrated its usefulness in treating malaria. It was likely astute observation rather than detailed modeling of disease that eventually provided patients with effective treatment for a serious disease. An equally remarkable example of rational therapy based on observation is that of medieval physicians who noticed that preparations of the French lilac reduced excess urine output in patients with diabetes mellitus. It was not until the twentieth century that these preparations were found to contain isoamylene guanidine, a substance that reduces blood sugar levels. The ability of guanidine to reduce blood sugar levels was itself discovered by happenstance, when researchers in 1918 discovered this effect while investigating the effect of guanidine in treating the side effects of parathyroidectomy. Guanidine can have some highly undesirable side effects but its effective use in diabetics led to the development of biguanides, medicines that are first line therapy for certain types of diabetes even in the twenty first century. What is remarkable is that the medieval physicians discovered an effective therapy with very little, if any, knowledge of the pathophysiology of the disease that they were treating.

This observation, trial-and-error approach to developing effective medical interventions is likely common to all forms of healing arts that have survived. Physicians from the time of Hippocrates (460-377 B.C.E.) observed the beneficial effects of treating wounds with wine and vinegar. The use of the latex of the opium poppy for pain relief dates back at least as far as recorded history, and the development of penicillin derived from Fleming's observation that mold contaminating a petri dish inhibited the growth of bacteria. The concept of hypothesizing a particular treatment and trying it out to see if it has a desirable effect was common both to the ancient practitioner who scoured for medicinal roots and plants, and to the modern pharmaceutical enterprise or university researcher who design therapies based on detailed models of biochemistry and molecular biology. The same process that led to the use of quinine as a treatment for malaria also produces the vast majority of new pharmacological agents. This incremental progress resulting from observation and experimentation is both beneficial and necessary since the intricate workings of the human body are far from completely understood.

Even the best sounding theories sometimes lead to therapies that do not pan out. It seems to make intuitive sense that preventing any type of heart rhythm disturbance would naturally reduce the occurrence of fatal rhythm disturbances. Modern medicine had therapies that suppressed abnormal heartbeats and it seemed to make almost conclusive sense that use of these agents would reduce the number of people who die of heart arrhythmias. When the theory was tried in actual people however, the exact opposite result was obtained. It is also common experience that therapies that prove effective in one person will fail to do so, or perhaps even be detrimental, in another. Many people had life saving experiences with penicillin; others had fatal allergic reactions. Some therapies, while having the desired result on the condition being treated cause their own associated mischief which are noted as undesirable side effects, such as nausea, rashes, hair loss, and kidney, liver and nerve damage.

It is undeniably true that modern western medicine and its historical and cultural counterparts developed therapies and interventions that are effective, at least for certain classes of ailments. This effectiveness is often limited both in duration and extent, and tempered by undesirable consequences. The potential benefit and precise role of medical therapies in human life are circumscribed by certain limiting principles. One of the most fundamental of such principles is that almost all medical and surgical therapies are approximations to the body's natural mechanisms for maintaining health. Therapies are not so much finely crafted keys that fit precisely with a given ailment, as much as crowbars that produce the same desired end as a key but do so far less elegantly and with potentially undesirable consequences. Paracelsus observed that all medicines are poisons, and that whether they caused or cured disease was a matter of dosing. Even completely successful surgical procedures do not leave the body in quite the same state it would have been in had the offending condition not been present. Removal of a diseased gall bladder may remove a source of infection and be an important step in restoring health, but the intervention nonetheless leaves the body without a gall bladder. Antibiotics kill invading pathogens through mechanisms that are completely different than that used by the immune system to accomplish the same end. Even when replacing deficient substances that are normally found within the body, such as insulin in the case of diabetes or thyroid hormone in the case of hypothyroidism, the exogenous replacement does not replicate the precise, continuous control produced by the body's own processes.

Medical therapies produce their effects in a variety of ways, many of which are poorly understood. Some interventions, such as antibiotics, work directly; others, such as the use of diuretics in heart failure, work by initiating a chain of responses that result in the desired effects. The mechanisms of other therapies are obscured by the fact that medicines producing opposite effects are used to treat the same condition. Brain injured patients often suffer from instability of their autonomic nervous system, producing symptoms such as rapid heartbeats, uncontrolled sweating and large swings in blood pressure. This condition is treated with medicines such as chlorpromazine, which antagonizes the action of the neurotransmitter dopamine, as well as bromocriptine, which instead produces dopamine-like effects. There are a great many interventions used in modern western medicine, both conventional and alternative, for which the precise manner in which they work is unknown.

Even placebos and sham treatments can appear effective in the appropriate environment. Many treatments are intended to reduce or relieve the symptoms accompanying some condition, and in these cases the treatment is effective solely if the patient perceives that it is. Therapies such as acupuncture, faith healing and shamanism may work in some cases simply because the approach of the practitioner is aligned with the needs of the patient. It is not necessary that the different models of disease and treatment contained within a particular healing art are objectively factual; it is only necessary that they lead to effective treatment. One such example from modern western medicine arises from the observation that high levels of inhaled oxygen leads to the retention of carbon dioxide in the blood of patients with severe emphysema. This led to the schematic model, familiar in medical schools and physician training programs, that the excess oxygen "suppresses the drive to breathe" of these patients, and served as a reminder to limit excessive oxygen use in this population. Even though the simple explanation does not describe the process by which oxygen produces high carbon dioxide levels in the blood, the model is still useful because it leads to appropriate medical interventions.

Modern medicine incorporates many therapies that seem to work despite their unintended effects on other body systems, undesirable side effects, or mechanisms that are arcane or altogether unknown. Some therapies, like antibiotics, work by augmenting the body's own functioning, while others, such as anti-inflammatory drugs and anticoagulants, work by opposing it. The body is remarkably forgiving of this lack of precision and conformity with nature's design, and this in fact suggests another of the unalterable principle of medical therapy: in order for any intervention to be ultimately successful, the body must have some reserve and ability to recover from the instant affliction. Voltaire claimed that the art of medicine consisted of amusing the patient while nature cured the disease, and while this likely overstates the case, it does serve as a reminder that modern medicine is only effective to the extent that a patient retains the capacity to improve. Surgeons will often refrain from operating on patients who are too sick to withstand the stresses of the procedure, and treatments such as dialysis and chemotherapy may be foregone if the patient is too debilitated to benefit from them.

Medical interventions aimed at improving the function of one organ often impose corresponding burdens on another. Treating congestive heart failure with diuretics, for example, often compromises function of the kidneys, and treating asthma with steroids provokes derangements in blood sugar control, blood pressure and bone metabolism. Often times a patient will present with two simultaneous conditions, the treatments of which antagonize each other. It is always frustrating for a physician to tend to a patient who has both a blood clot on the lung and a bleeding ulcer, or one whose blood pressure is dangerously low but who also has fluid on his lungs. In the latter case, giving fluids might improve the blood pressure but worsen the patient's lung function. These examples serve to highlight the notion that medical interventions are not faithful replacements for the abnormal functions that they are designed to treat. Successful therapy requires a compatible interaction between the treatment and the bodily processes that permit or produce healing.

The medical art is complicated by the fact that the same intervention may produce different outcomes in different patients. A blood thinner that prevents blood clots from causing strokes in one patient may cause a brain hemorrhage in another. Furthermore, a therapy that works well in a particular patient may have decreasing effectiveness over time. A reality of medical treatment is that the body may respond to it in ways that are inconvenient to the aims of the patient and practitioner. Many therapies produce extraordinary benefits in the short term and cause deleterious effects over longer periods. Steroids used to treat exacerbations of autoimmune diseases or asthma often lead to prompt relief of symptoms, but if continued over time can cause bone loss, weight gain, thinning of the skin and easy bruising, cataracts, diabetes and undesirable psychological effects. Antibiotics may be quite effective initially, but repeated exposures may encourage the emergence of drug resistance by infecting organisms. Diuretics may become less effective over time as the body adapts to their mechanisms of action. Occasionally the opposite course ensues, and interventions that initially produce deterioration in the patient's condition result in long-term benefits. It was observed initially that the class of blood pressure drugs known as beta-blockers worsened the symptoms of heart failure, and thus should be avoided in patients with that condition. Subsequent investigation revealed however, that beta-blockers preserve the health of the heart muscle and are beneficial as long-term treatment.

This time-dependent effect of medical therapies mirrors the body's response to changes in condition or environment. The body frequently has an acute response that rapidly compensates for a given change, but that is deleterious when activated chronically. One example of this phenomenon is the kidney's response to an injury that reduces the amount of specialized tissue available for filtering the blood. The kidney's initial response to this circumstance is to increase the pressure at which the remaining tissue filters the blood, which increases the rate of filtration per amount of tissue. This results in partial compensation for the lost function, but over time the increased pressure damages the remaining tissue, leading to further loss of function. Another example concerns the body's response to acute heart failure. Compromised heart function leads to stimulation of the heart muscle by adrenaline, which improves the efficiency of heart and relieves symptoms. Over time however, long-term stimulation by adrenaline has deleterious effects on heart muscle and results in progressive decline. This is why blocking the effects of adrenaline with beta-blockers causes initial worsening of symptoms, but provides longer-term benefit.

The experience of treating illness and injury with various interventions and medicines demonstrates that such interventions are seldom curative or even effective by themselves. Successful treatment entails an interaction between the body and the therapy, and quite often between the body and the therapist. The body is often able to accommodate stressful or injudicious therapies, and often times returns to health as much in spite of as because of the interventions to which it is subjected. While rational therapy and modern western medicine attempt to tailor specific treatments to particular ailments, the simple truth is that the systems and process used by the body to maintain health and function are not always amenable to these treatments. The body was not designed for all of the interventions that modern medicine makes available to it. One example of this concept concerns surgery. It is quite reasonable to assume that the body's response to penetrating trauma, which is what surgery is, did not account for the possibility that such trauma was therapeutic. Thus, the natural response to invasion by a foreign object, or disruption of the integrity of the circulatory system, is to dispose the blood to form clots to stop the bleeding. This is quite a reasonable and likely effective response when penetrating trauma was the result of wounds inflicted by wild animals or bellicose neighbors, but the tendency to clot is a nuisance for modern treatments such as surgery for joint replacement, or the replacement of damaged heart valves. The body's well-intended, and in fact well designed, contingency for invasion by sharp objects often frustrates modern medical procedures and must be accommodated by using anti-clotting medicines. Likewise the body's response to the presence of invading biological tissue, which is what an organ transplant is, is to mobilize the immune system against it. Successful therapy in these cases requires suppression of the immune system, with the increased risk of serious infection that such treatment entails.

Perhaps the most poignant example of a mismatch between the effects of modern medicine and the body's natural processes is that in which medical intervention keeps the body alive long after the mind has significantly declined. There are likely sound teleological reasons why the cells of the central nervous system do not regenerate once destroyed. It may be that such a strategy is necessary to the processing of external information, the ability to distinguish between real and imagined experiences, and the processing of memory. It may perhaps be a defense against the development of tumors in highly metabolically active tissue, or it may simply be an accident of evolution. Whatever the case, the decline of cognitive functioning in the elderly is very common and its prevalence increases markedly with age. It should be expected that at one time the expected life span of a person's higher cognitive functioning was at least as long as the expected duration of his or her life. This is no longer reliably the case due to modern medical interventions such as cardiac stents, hemodialysis, organ transplants, and highly effective treatments for diabetes and cancer. It is no longer a rare experience that a person may long outlive his cognitive function. This is another example of the principle that modern medicine often involves consequences beyond the effectiveness of a particular therapy.

The effectiveness of therapy is simply one facet of the healing arts. Health is a desired end but healing is a process, one that often consumes a large portion of an individual's life. Even if health is not ultimately achieved, the interaction between practitioner and patient is often a valuable, meaningful experience for both parties. Modern medicine presents several challenges to this notion. Modern technology often makes the process of diagnosis and treatment impersonal, or too dismissive of the subjective needs of the patient, in deference to scientific data. Initiatives that have as their goal increased efficiency in the use of resources or standardization of therapies can create a barrier to a deeply therapeutic relationship. Increasing specialization diffuses the care among several providers, which may maximize available expertise at the expense of more intimate interactions. These issues may be natural consequences of processes that lead to better clinical outcome and more efficient use of medical resources, but they may simultaneously represent regrettable losses of substance from the human element of medicine.

The idea that the interaction between patient and practitioner is an important element in the healing arts is probably as old as medicine itself. Plato, in Book IV of his *Laws*, in making a point regarding legislation, remarked:

> And did you ever observe that there are two classes of patients in states, slaves and freemen; and the slave doctors run about and cure the slaves, or wait for them in the dispensaries-practitioners of this sort never talk to their patients individually, or let them talk about their own individual complaints? The slave doctor prescribes what mere experience suggests, as if he had exact knowledge; and when he has given his orders, like a tyrant, he rushes off with equal assurance to some other servant who is ill; and so he relieves the master of the house of the care of

his invalid slaves. But the other doctor, who is a freeman, attends and practices upon freemen; and he carries his enquiries far back, and goes into the nature of the disorder; he enters into discourse with the patient and with his friends, and is at once getting information from the sick man, and also instructing him as far as he is able, and he will not prescribe for him until he has first convinced him; at last, when he has brought the patient more and more under his persuasive influences and set him on the road to health, he attempts to effect a cure.

A trusting relationship between patient and provider would seem to be desirable, if for no other reason than the patient is more likely to participate in and comply with therapy that he believes will be beneficial. This is particularly so because therapies often cause side effects, discomfort or involve periods of discouraging trial. In such circumstances, a trusting relationship between the patient and practitioner is essential. Centuries of experience have shown that the processes of diagnosis and prescribing require knowledge of facts and symptoms that a patient would not share with acquaintances, or perhaps even family. Successful therapy often involves providing the patient with insights that are not likely to emerge from an impersonal discussion of a few common symptoms. In addition, experience suggests that the process of healing from an injury or recovering from ill health is facilitated by conveying a sense that someone cares about relieving the patient's suffering and is concerned about the patient as a person. It is no slight to physicians to observe that the majority of actual patient care in hospitals is provided by the nurses who interact with the patient many times during the day and night, whose attention provides comfort, and who create the environment in which patients convalesce, and endure the crises in their diseases.

There is something therapeutic in a demonstration of concern, but while it is expected that those caring for and attempting to treat a particular patient convey a sense of caring, there are practical limits to this process. A practitioner is expected to maintain a professional detachment from the experience of his or her patient. Therapeutic relationships involve a measure of objectivity, and this is compromised when the healer identifies too closely with the suffering of the patient. This is why family members do not serve on juries, either when they are related to victim or accused. It is also why physicians generally avoid diagnosing the diseases of, and treating the illnesses of family members except in extraordinary circumstances. Objectivity on the part of the physician or other practitioner is necessary to sound judgment and to protect therapeutic decisions from being adversely influenced by emotion. There is always a risk that the denial in which some patients seek refuge from the consequences of their afflictions will also affect those physicians who have come to sympathize too closely with them. Cold, rational analysis often provides the resolution of a clinical mystery where close affectionate attention is, by itself, insufficient.

Modern medicine presents a number of impediments to forming appropriate therapeutic relationships between those who suffer and those who attempt to treat them. These impediments are sometimes unavoidable and simply represent reasonable trade-offs necessary to attain some other benefit to be found in a particular relationship. Sometimes the impediment arises from the complexity of the systems associated with modern medicine; sometimes they are the product of poorly thought-out policies.

One phenomenon that can impair the development of a thorough practitioner-patient relationship is the increasing prevalence of specialization in medical knowledge and treatment. Specialization in healthcare is not a recent development and the ancient Greek historian Herodotus described the specialization of medical care in ancient Egypt:

> Medicine is practiced among them on a plan of separation; each physician treats a single disorder and no more; thus the country swarms with

> medical practitioners, some undertaking to cure diseases of the eye, others of the hand, others again of the teeth, others of the intestines and some of those which are not local.

Specialization has the potential to provide significant benefits to modern healthcare, primarily by increasing the efficiency of services and permitting patients to access expertise beyond that which may be possessed by a general practitioner. Specialization has provided well-demonstrated benefits in the area of economics, where Leonard E. Read showed that without it, it would be unlikely that anyone could produce something as simple as a pencil. Many disciplines require years of dedicated study to master, and specialization is therefore necessary to access many of the more complex therapies. A radiologist typically spends four to five years honing the art of interpreting medical images, and can thus provide a service to patients that is beyond the experience of the generalist, whose time and education are spread across much wider areas. Surgeons who specialize in the nervous system or vascular abnormalities also have years of training beyond that necessary to show competence in basic surgical technique.

Expertise that a specialist brings to the care of a patient often comes at the expense of a deeper relationship. It is often the case that a generalist, once having localized the source of complaint, will refer the patient to a specialist in the area of concern. The specialist will then focus on the subject of his own expertise, brooding over the proper course of therapy but leaving to others the broader details that affect the patient's health. Just as a generalist must necessarily devote his time to a broad spectrum of medical knowledge, which limits his ability to aggressively focus on any one area, the specialist must concentrate on his own area of expertise to the neglect of others. Since the care of a particular patient may be shared among multiple specialists, each providing valuable and unique expertise, it should not be expected that any of them could develop the same bond that might exist between that patient and a single generalist who takes the time to learn the details of the patient's life over time, and over a variety of maladies.

Relationships that involve deep understanding of the patient's circumstances and background are also inhibited by the prevalence of medical technology. In some respects this is understandable and perhaps even inevitable. The diagnostic information that previously involved becoming familiar with the patient's history, symptoms, habits and friends can now be somewhat replaced by technology that probes directly at the biological and pathogenic processes that are responsible for the patient's complaint. People trust science because science has a track record, and it is a natural consequence that sometimes they may trust in science more than the human provider who undertakes to treat their illness. A physician who correctly sifts and deciphers disparate scraps of physical exam findings and the patient's own descriptions of his symptoms may impress, but the detailed images of a magnetic resonance imaging scan can awe.

The institutions and intertwined entities that make up the modern healthcare system also interpose between patients and practitioners of the healing arts. Insurance companies, through their provider panels, often dictate which providers a patient can see. Hospital administrators may encourage physicians to use expensive and lucrative technologies when there is a source of payment, and forego them when there is not. Pharmaceutical firms that market directly to patients, popular media that encourage suspicion toward the motives and conflicted interests of medical providers, and friends and family who may proselytize for novel theories or trendy cures all undermine the relationship between physician and patient.

Sometimes the physician patient relationship is affected by well-intentioned and even well executed efforts to improve patient care. While the typical example of medical decision-making involves a practitioner using informed judgment to direct therapy, it is increasingly the case that the patient's care may have been decided by remote experts who never see the patient or follow the individual consequences of their work. Medical care is increasingly scrutinized against guidelines, benchmarks, clinical pathways and performance standards that are intended to improve the use of evidence in patient care, but which have the attendant effect of subjecting a patient to therapy that was designed for a population of patients, with which he may have only a minimum in common. Many conditions, such as chest pain are now treated largely by algorithms that increase the likelihood that a patient experiencing a heart attack is provided with what is considered the appropriate standard of care. The treatment is nonetheless prescribed by a committee trying to address the needs of patients generally, but those patients may differ significantly from each other in their ailments and needs.

The success of a particular form of therapy is influenced by more than the subtleties of that therapy, a condition that is responsive to it, and an appropriate relationship with the practitioner who provides it. Success also depends upon the purpose for which a remedy is sought. Considerations upon which therapeutic decisions are based often include matters outside of the patient and the malady. Sometimes treatment is provided for the benefit of persons other than the patient who receives them. Physicians often feel compelled to order diagnostic studies or initiate treatment in order to assuage the anxieties of a family member. Likewise, treatment is often provided, not because a physician suspects that a patient has a particular condition, but because the patient simply worries that he might.

Although seldom identified as such, medical therapy is often a prop in dramatic scenes that play out during medical crises, or when patients near the end of life. It is not uncommon for treatment to proceed according to idealistic assumptions that the patient may recover from metastatic cancer or a devastating stroke, even when common sense and the clinical evidence indicate otherwise. Treatment is sometimes provided to stave off the realization that not all diseases have a remedy, or as a form of affirmation that the provider has something to offer. This may be one reason why antibiotics, for example, are sometimes prescribed for conditions where one would not expect them to provide a benefit. In such cases, it is helpful if the patient presents with a condition that will get better on its own anyway. Sometimes providing treatment or medicines is little more than an expression of optimism that things might get better.

Therapy is not the end point of modern medicine, or really any type of healing art. It is a part of a process by which healers assist patients through the challenges presented by illness and injury. Therapies do not always work; sometimes they make things worse; but they remain the most tangible part of a very human instinct, and that is to defy the inevitability of decline and suffering and to continue to live meaningful life despite the frailties to which human beings are subject.

5

ETHICS

Everyone's life is exposed to injury, disease and the healing arts to one degree or another. Even if a specific person does not experience these directly, it is almost certain that he or she will have a family member or close acquaintance who will. For this reason, healthcare impacts everyone's life, and the conduct of those that undertake to provide healthcare to others should be subject to certain guiding principles.

Human life is subject to threats and burdens that arise from nature and conflicting interests, and human beings developed institutions like medicine, the law, government, and military organizations in order to address them. For these institutions to be effective they must be able to significantly affect people's lives and, as a result, can do so in ways that are both positive and negative. Good medicine, good government and good laws have positive influences in human life and bad medicine, government or law causes significant suffering and misery. In each case, reason, conscience and some sense of duty must distinguish between conduct that makes institutions beneficial and that which causes harm. Institutions like medicine, which can produce enormous benefits or cause great harm, must be constrained by ethical principles if they are to benefit both individual people and societies in general.

Ethics, like medicine itself, developed and persists because it is useful. It is reasonable to assume that even the most primitive of men noticed that some actions were attended by desirable consequences, while others were the source of pain and regret. The processes of observation and analysis would have led to the notion that some actions were good and others bad. It should not have required consultation with a philosopher to understand that behaving in a certain way was associated with living better, and that some conduct should be avoided because, even if it provided a short term benefit in an individual case, it was not consistent with those identified principles that were understood to be part of a good life.

There are several characteristics of the healing arts that make ethics essential. One of the most fundamental of these is that illness and injury naturally make patients vulnerable to the ulterior interests of those from whom they seek help. There is often a disparity in knowledge about the condition of concern, making it necessary for the patient to trust the practitioner. This trust can be abused by the unscrupulous or self-interested. Even if they do not trust the provider, patients may have no realistic option other than to submit to the diagnostic procedures and therapies that the provider prescribes. Persons afflicted with injuries and disease are often vulnerable because of the psychological responses to their conditions. Those who are ill, as well as their families, are often influenced by fear, hope, despair, anger and denial. As a result, they may be swayed by appeals that would be considered irrational in less urgent circumstances. Because of this, the perception that a healer can provide comfort and cure diseases can be used to exploit patients and their families, and a credible system of providing healthcare must develop ethical restraints that discourage such mischief.

Ethical boundaries are also necessary because the art and science of medicine, like all technologies, have no inherent morality, and can be used for either beneficent or malign purposes. Activities of medically trained personnel during the Second World War, such as the human experiments conducted by Josef Mengele in Nazi Germany and the germ warfare studies performed in Northeastern

China at Imperial Japan's Unit 731 provide sobering examples of this fact. Similarly, the use of psychiatric techniques to the detriment of political prisoners and prisoners of conscience in the Soviet Union, and the non-consensual syphilis experiments undertaken under government auspices in Tuskegee, Alabama illustrate the dark consequences that can occur when medicine is practiced in a manner in which the welfare of the patient is subordinated to other interests.

Medical science has progressed to the point where it can produce outcomes that were once impossible, but which we are not yet sure if they are desirable or appropriate. Medical advances have forced practically continuous re-evaluation of what parts of human life, if any, should be beyond human interference. We have, for some time, been in an age where outcomes may be pursued simply because they are possible without regard to how they affect more philosophical concerns of whether they are humane, dignified, or consistent with the enlightened concepts of how human beings should treat each other.

The inescapable reality that makes ethics indispensable to modern medicine is that the healthcare of a particular patient involves many, often competing, interests. Healthcare is now so complex and involves so many disparate components that the concept of a patient and practitioner deciding between the two of them how they will manage an injury or illness is a quaint abstraction. The reality is now that there are financial, regulatory, public policy, cultural, business, and myriad other concerns that encroach upon individual healthcare decisions. A physician treating a patient for pneumonia can expect to be reminded of not only the patient's interests, but also those of the hospital, patient's insurance company, nursing staff, pharmaceutical company, patient's family, state licensing board, professional societies, etc. The proponents of each of these interests will explicitly demur that everyone "wants what is best for the patient" but this is not always the case in practice. Practically no one wants what is best for the patient, including often the patient. Patients frequently refuse therapy that they consider too burdensome, painful, costly, or uncomfortable. The fact that quitting smoking is what seems best for the patient does not always translate into healthier habits. Instead, what nearly all parties to healthcare decisions want is what is good enough for the patient, considering his or her own interests.

Hospitals want to provide adequate care consistent with their staffing abilities, and need to recoup investments in expensive technologies. They want physicians to practice in such a way that makes demonstrating regulatory compliance easier. They want the care of patients to accommodate often-irrational reimbursement constraints imposed by remote functionaries. Insurance companies want adequate treatment in line with prudent actuarial practice; pharmaceutical companies want physicians to consider their products; nursing staffs want the physician's orders to be mindful that there are other patients that need care, and just because something sounds trivial or mundane does not mean that it turns out that way in practice. The physician may have his or her own interests, such as financial incentives to pursue a particular course of therapy, or keep the patient under treatment for an extended period, or he may be concerned about liability issues that result in defensive medicine being practiced upon the patient. Patient's families may demand unhelpful testing simply to reassure themselves that some feared condition is not lurking beyond the notice of the physician, or demand what is otherwise objectively futile care because they are not yet ready to accept the inevitable.

Varying interests and conflicts of interests challenge the priorities of the practitioner, necessitating reference to some established framework for preserving the traditional obligations of the practitioner in treating ill or injured patients. Medical ethics tends to fall into two broad, if somewhat arbitrary classes: aspirational and practical. The practical ethics is that which address observable actions that reason and experience indicate are necessary to the effective practice of healing arts. These include guidance for issues such as patient confidentiality, which is necessary to permit open and frank communication between patient and provider. Another is avoidance of obvious self-dealing on the part of the practitioner, or allowing an unqualified person to practice upon the patient. Because compliance with the practical ethical constraints is observable and verifiable, they are often the subjects of explicit regulation; thus there are formal regulations pertaining to patient privacy, physician self-referral, and the unlicensed practice of medicine.

As with many other objects of regulation, the healing arts provide a robust substrate for unintended consequences, inefficiency and anomalous results. Regulations of general application, by their very nature are difficult to conform to the unique circumstances of particular cases. The officials that promulgate regulations, including those that codify certain ethical considerations related to healthcare, often view their mandates and prohibitions as floors relative to acceptable conduct, whereas those charged with complying with those regulations often view them as ceilings, i.e. the most that regulators can expect. In such circumstances compliance with the regulations imposes another competing interest into the decision-making for an individual patient, not always to that patient's benefit.

Even though codifying ethical considerations into explicit regulations may be accompanied by some drawbacks, it is not surprising that such regulations exist. Considering the importance of healthcare to functioning societies, and the great harm that can occur when it is misused, it is both understandable and necessary for those societies to exert some control over what is and is not acceptable healthcare behavior.

The second class of ethical constraints is that which concerns the idea of medicine as a noble profession, and which embraces such virtues as compassion, empathy and humane regard for the dignity of human life. The effects of these ethical concerns are not readily observable, and thus cannot be easily enforced by external regulation. They affect and determine the actions of practitioners who are confronted with conflicting interests, when motivations and priorities are not explicit. The situations in which such ethical principles influence medical decision making may include, for example, the situations where what the practitioner and patient decide is the best course of action is contrary to accepted norms, or the case where the demands of the family are contrary to an incapacitated patient's values. In such cases there is no "right answer," and no clearly understood action that is demonstrably contrary to an objective understanding of good medicine. The sense that a conflict exists may not even be apparent to anyone but the practitioner involved. Similar circumstances may lead to different courses of action for different patients, simply because the values and interests of those patients differ.

Another source of conflict in a physician's obligations arises from the fact that healthcare is a limited resource. Physicians and other providers are expected to be stewards of the healthcare system, and this can potentially place them in conflict with the interests of their patients. Physicians are expected to limit the use of antibiotic therapies so as to impede the development of antibiotic resistance, to forego expensive diagnostic studies and marginally effective therapies to protect the solvency of stressed healthcare systems, and to be cost-conscious in even the most effective treatment. Sometimes the effects on patients are subtle, such as using a less expensive medicine that has a higher incidence of side effects, or one that must be given more frequently. Sometimes the choices are between more obviously disparate alternatives, such as when an extensive and traumatic surgical technique is selected over more expensive, but less invasive options. These conflicts can become particularly uncomfortable when the alteration in a patient's care inures to the benefit of shareholders of for-profit businesses, rather than to an entity whose interests are more observably altruistic.

Because various interests compete for consideration in medical decision-making, it is necessary for the practitioner who provides therapy to be able to prioritize among them. The seemingly obvious approach of placing the patient's interests first does not always provide practical guidance however. Patients may be unsure of exactly what their interest is, as when a cancer patient has difficulty choosing between aggressive treatment with little or no hope of cure, or being made as comfortable as possible. Patients may struggle with allegiances to their own desires, and the feelings of family or religious teachings. They may have requests that are ethically disquieting for the physician, such as for euthanasia, excessive prescriptions for narcotics, or unnecessary therapies. A physician may have to rely on the word of a surrogate decision-maker whose own wishes and goals of treatment, even if well intentioned, conflict with those of the patient. The patient's own consideration of his or her interests and values may be affected by denial, unrealistic expectations, or motives having little to do with healthcare issues. Patients may reject potentially curative therapy because they fear attendant side effects, or because it is too expensive. Putting the patient's interest first is not always straightforward, or even possible, because of difficulty defining what that interest is, and because that interest may compete with other interests that are accorded higher priority.

Not every healthcare related interest of a patient is compatible with broader social interests. It is certainly understandable that a drug addict may be interested in receiving opioid pain medications, seeking short-term relief from the consequences of his addiction, but this conflicts with other societal values regarding the proper use of such medications.

Medicine and other healing arts are elements of human life that must exist with other interests in a society. The health concerns of a particular individual do not confer upon that individual the right to subordinate the competing interests of others. In many instances, practitioners must decide the priority of competing legitimate interests, and this includes his or her own. A physician may be confronted with a patient who he feels he can no longer treat because the patient does not follow treatment recommendations. Another physician may decide that ordering pointless and futile therapies for a terminal patient in deference to the family's wishes is wrong, even when the opposite conclusion represents the path of least resistance.

The decisions that implicate aspirational ethics leave no tell-tale evidence of ethical lapses. At worst they appear to be judgment calls for which improper motives might be suspected, but not proven. For this reason, these types of ethical dilemmas require practitioners to have some manner of a well-formed conscience. The inherent duty that arises from a healer undertaking to treat a patient in such a manner that the undertaking is virtuous ultimately requires integrity on the part of the practitioner.

Medicine cannot survive either as an institution, or the more abstract "noble profession," unless it is practiced by at least some people who are influenced by notions of right and wrong. The physician or other healing practitioner is a moral agent, and is responsible for the consequences of his or her conduct, even when that conduct is in the interests of a patient. Matters of conscience may legitimately trump even life and death concerns for the patient. While the patient's health, and what is done to his body are properly viewed as subjective and personal, healthcare must be provided by others, in circumstances that implicate the rights and values of persons outside the physician patient relationship.

Successful societies necessarily demand some concessions from their members and sometimes those concessions affect medical decisions. It is inevitable that individual values will occasionally conflict with broader societal values, and this conflict will sometimes present an ethical quandary for the practitioner. Medical decisions throughout much of history were guided by the principle of paternalism; the notion that the practitioner would use his or her superior knowledge and skill to do what was best for the patient. This principle presupposed some standard by which to determine what was "best," and gradually the concept evolved that the person who knew what was best for the patient was the patient. The principle of paternalism gave way, at least technically, to the concept of patient autonomy. Paternalism seems to be based on the assumption that there is an objective measure of what is best for the patient, and that the practitioner has the requisite background and knowledge to identify it and apply it in a given case. Patient autonomy, on the other hand, presumes that what is best is ultimately a subjective, rather than objective determination, and even if an objective standard is used, the patient should have some say in its application. The distinction between paternalism and patient autonomy has other dimensions as well. Paternalism does not depend so much on the existence of some identifiable, objective measure of what the patient's interests should be, rather, it subordinates the values of the patient to what are ultimately cultural values.

Issues of human reproduction, use of medical resources, care of the mentally ill and use of medical interventions for reasons other than to treat specific disease states naturally intersect with medical decision making. It was cultural values rather than isolated medical considerations that disfavored artificial birth control, abortion, incarcerating the mentally ill, and restricting the use of certain drugs. Even today, proscriptions against euthanasia, abortion for sex selection and selling one's own kidney for transplant, are more reflections of prevailing cultural norms than expressions of what individual patients would subjectively recognize as desirable.

While paternalism provides one vehicle for integrating cultural values into individual medical decisions, explicit rejection of that doctrine does not thereby preclude such values from those decisions. Cultural and societal values are inherent in healthcare decisions, and societal institutions ensure that they are considered. If societies do not endorse paternalism as an effective principle for promoting their interests, they construct other institutions for the same purpose. Societies that ration care according to the pronouncements of some body of experts subordinate "what is best for the patient" to those considerations better served by rationing. Even in situations without such an explicit and transparent process, when expert panels, clinical guidelines, and treatment algorithms influence care, those devices are influenced by broader concerns, and are often promulgated explicitly to address those concerns.

Another way in which societal values influence individual medical decisions is through the use of surrogate, and often quite abstract goals of therapy. A common example of such a goal is "quality of life." It is common for medical providers to balk at sophisticated and expensive therapy for a severely disabled patient by focusing not upon the actual intended result of that therapy, i.e. keeping the patient alive, but upon the more subjective and value-laden concept of "quality."

What practitioners of the healing arts should or should not do in particular cases often involves consideration of unique circumstances and therefore resists application of general rules and broad principles. While it is desirable that there be some articulable principles guiding the conduct of physicians and other practitioners, attempts to comprehensively codify these principles can provide only the crudest of guidance. Perhaps the most well known of such attempts is what is commonly referred to as the Hippocratic oath, which is popularly understood to contain the admonition, *primum, non nocere*, or "first, do no harm." The most obvious characteristic of this directive is that it is incompatible with the practice of modern medicine. If a surgeon were strictly to adhere to this precept, he would never be tempted to the operating room after advising the patient of the potential risks and benefits of surgery. Risk is inherent in medicine. Medical and surgical interventions affect the way the body works and is put together; it is unreasonable to expect that such interventions would not occasionally harm an organism as complex and variable as the human body. Anyone who has seen an open heart surgery patient wheeled into the recovery room, sedated on a ventilator, with vital signs managed by a cocktail of intravenous medicines dripping into his body would have a hard time ignoring that some harm was done. In the particular case, as well as similar cases such as amputation, it is recognized that the harm done is a reasonable trade off for the expected therapeutic benefit.

The admonition to do no harm was not part of an oath written by Hippocrates. The wording is contained in Book I of his work *Epidemics*, in which he stated "The physician must be able to tell the antecedents, know the present, and foretell the future - must mediate these things, and have two special objects in view with regard to disease, namely, to do good or to do no harm." The classical version of the oath contained the somewhat more practical pledge "I will follow that system of regimen which, according to my ability and judgment, I consider for the benefit of my patients, and abstain from whatever is deleterious and mischievous." The first recorded administration of the oath to medical school graduates occurred in Holland in 1508. The classical version of the oath contained explicit rejection of both euthanasia and abortion, but it has been tweaked and adapted to conform to cultural and social values over time. These alterations follow directly from the premise that the physician does not treat patients in a vacuum, isolated from extrinsic considerations and values. In the modern era, the Oath of Hippocrates is a useful reminder that the vast power and effectiveness of medical science can be used with both good intentions as well as bad, and that those who undertake to treat injury and disease are responsible for the moral consequences of their practice.

Medicine has always been capable of doing harm as well as good. This inescapable fact has not been affected by technological advances or the maturing of institutions that comprise the healing arts. In some instances, these have made the avoidance of harm more of a challenge. Modern medicine has begotten circumstances in which it is difficult to tell whether intervention has produced a good outcome or a bad one. An example of such a case is that in which a severely brain injured, comatose patient is kept alive indefinitely, with necessary functions being provided by dialysis machines and mechanical ventilators. Even when the effect is exactly that which was intended, the limits of medical science sometimes leave patients stranded in a type of purgatory between their underlying infirmities and the desired results that medicine cannot quite provide. Science sometimes promises that which it cannot deliver, and it puts those who rely on such promises at risk. In such circumstances, it is the ethical guideposts of the practitioner that provide the defense against harm.

The ability, or even the perception of the ability, of the healing arts to affect the health of individual people has consequences that extend beyond the interaction between physician and patient. The perception that medicine is the last line of defense against devastating plagues, that it can mend lives and return patients to contributing members of society, and at least partially alleviate the harsh consequences of what otherwise appears to be random misfortune makes it a societal asset. The notion that medicine can have both beneficial and harmful effects in people's lives produces secondary concerns as to how societies regulate and control healthcare.

One of the most fundamental of these societal concerns is whether all people should have equal access to healthcare services, or whether services that cannot be available to all should be denied to all; in other words, is healthcare a right? The simple question tends to provoke of frenzy of semantic parsing; what is meant by each of the terms, healthcare and right? Is "right" intended in the legal sense, as a sentimental aspiration, or as a philosophical abstraction? If healthcare is a right, is the obligation of government simply to refrain from enacting barriers to specific therapies, or is it more in the sense of an affirmative obligation to ensure that such therapies are provided? Likewise, does the word "healthcare" encompass only the non-controversial treatment of commonly accepted injuries and diseases, or does it extend to interventions solely to advance the personal preferences and perceptions of specific patients?

If one were to defer the more abstract philosophical and legalistic attributes of rights and confine analysis to empiric observation, healthcare is not a right. It is not one in the sense that society must refrain from constructing impediments to particular therapies, and it is not one in the sense that there is an affirmative obligation to provide it. Examples of the former proposition are readily observed: states regulate who can provide medical treatment, and place requirements on how particular therapies can be delivered. Some therapies are banned altogether. Societies determined that the beneficial, pain relieving affects of diamorphine, more commonly known as heroin, were outweighed by other factors. As a result, many patients do not have a right to medicinal use of heroin. Societies do not allow an unlimited access to medical therapies, because medical interventions can be harmful as well as beneficial, and societies need not defer the avoidance of harm solely to the discretion of the practitioner. Practitioners, like the therapies they provide, can be both good and bad, and societies have an interest in mitigating the undesirable results of the latter.

Healthcare is also not a right in the sense that there is an affirmative obligation to provide it to anyone who has need of it. This is simply because healthcare is a service that must be provided by others, and no one has a claim of right to the labor or services of another without that other person's consent. Despite this, there is a natural sympathy for the proposition that healthcare, like food and shelter, are simply components of a fundamental right to life. As much appeal as this argument has, however, it is false. The analogy between food and healthcare breaks down over the point of necessity. Food is necessary to the survival of everyone; healthcare, while inarguably essential to the lives of certain individuals is not necessary to human life in general.

Regarding healthcare as a right introduces difficulties into the concept of rights as commonly understood. This is so because of ambiguity and a debilitating laxity in the meaning of the term "healthcare." It is problematic to declare something a right and then after the fact define what that something is. A decent respect for the concept of rights requires those claims and freedoms that are regarded as rights to possess identifiable qualities worthy of the appellation, not simply bear a cosmetic resemblance to something else that is recognized as a right. "Healthcare" encompasses a large number of items, some necessary to treat injuries and diseases and some not. Some things that are referred to generically as healthcare are beneficial to some people and irrelevant or even harmful to others. Some people use substances that have medicinal benefits for non-medicinal reasons, such as recreation, or to enhance athletic performance. Others desire surgical interventions for elective reasons unrelated to any identifiable disease or injury, such as elective cosmetic procedures, or interventions to abrogate fertility. Sometimes interventions that are commonly regarded as healthcare are harmful, frivolous or extravagant. It is problematic to confer the same moral or legal status on interventions that have purely subjective or idiosyncratic benefits as we do to medical therapies that have a more objective benefit simply because they share a common origin.

Even if healthcare were to be considered a right in the abstract sense, there are practical limitations to treating it as such. While healthcare may be viewed as a right or an entitlement from the perspective of the recipient, it is a limited resource when viewed from that of the providers. There is no practical method by which to limit the demand for healthcare to the ability to provide it; the consequence of which is rationing of or denial of healthcare to some who seek it. This circumstance is not compatible with the popular notions of rights, especially that which considers healthcare an entitlement. The potential that demand for healthcare services might outstrip supply is contrary to the notion of healthcare as a right. It is anomalous, and rather pointless to assert that people enjoy a right to something that practical considerations dictate that they cannot have.

Whether or not one considers healthcare a right, there is a natural sympathy for the idea that access to at least some basic healthcare should not be denied solely because of financial poverty, social status or personal beliefs. This idea does not originate with any single specific consideration, such as justice or fairness, rather it arises from the notion of what obligations societies must assume in order to thrive and prosper. An obligation to provide healthcare, at least in prescribed circumstances, arises from the values that a society adopts in order to enable opportunities for happiness and meaningful life for its members. This is not a novel concept, and is familiar throughout history as the virtue of charity. It may be taken as given that the experience of charity benefits all parties concerned. It cannot escape notice how many hospitals (and universities and homeless shelters) bear the name of some saint or religion or philanthropist or charitable guild. Charity is a virtue that recognizes that human life has as intrinsic value apart from affluence or political connection. It is a natural expression of compassion and the human empathy that is necessary for people to coexist and pursue happiness amongst their neighbors. Charitable societies may be expected to be more successful than less generous ones because they would presumably be more cognizant of the interdependence and synergistic relationships among their members. Societies typically undertake to provide a certain measure of healthcare, such as emergency services, based only on the patient's status as a human being, because to do so is a reflection of common human decency, individual empathy and an enlightened view of civilized behavior.

Charity does not require government intervention to be effective. It arises from the virtue of individual people, and it depends upon them for its maintenance. A collection of misers is unlikely to form a generous mob. The benefits that societies enjoy from charity derive from the virtue and decency of individual people, rather than as a byproduct of some policy. The charity that is representative of a civilized and decent society is that which is voluntary and arises from authentic concern for fellow humans. Those who receive healthcare services simply because of need do so not because they are entitled to those services or have a right to them, but because others are virtuous enough to provide them.

Somehow the concept of charity has become offensive and it has become associated with a stigma of helplessness or failure on the part of those who receive it. There is now an intellectual fashion of addressing this stigma by cloaking what is otherwise a very basic expression of human kindness and concern in government programs and euphemisms. It is natural for decent people to provide care to those without means to provide their own; it is natural for decent recipients of such care to be grateful for it, and both are necessary to the progress of societies composed of people whose circumstances and fortunes vary widely. Charity is not an asset to a society because it is a mechanism to distribute resources; its value lies in the shared kindnesses, the reciprocated thoughtfulness and the genuine concern for others that people need in order to live amongst one another. It may matter little to an individual of limited means whether he receives care because the resources necessary to provide it were willingly donated or forcibly confiscated, but such a distinction does matter to the bonds that hold societies together.

There are very real consequences to the distinction between entitlement and charity, not the least of which is that the former ultimately involves force and the latter does not. This same attribute may make entitlements more predictable than reliance on charitable good will, but does so by altering the relationship between society and those who comprise it, and between those whose resources are used to provide benefits and those who receive them. A society that provides for the less fortunate by forcibly confiscating the resources of others occupies a different moral orbit than one in which such provision results from altruism. Coerced virtue is not really virtuous, and it is the more genuine variety that is essential to those higher qualities to which human beings naturally aspire.

There is also a practical aspect to distinguishing between voluntary charity and mandated entitlement. Inherent in the concept of entitlement is the concept of permanence, or at least relative permanence. This is in fact one of the attractive attributes of viewing healthcare services as entitlements; they are not likely to disappear as such on a whim. The same property that makes their existence more or less permanent also makes them resistant to change and adaptation. The same considerations that make recipients resistant to changes in access to promised services also makes them resistant to changes in the methods and substance of those services, even when these become obsolete. Predictability is sometimes the adversary of efficiency. Those that freely donate their assets for the benefit of others have an incentive to develop and adopt newer and better methods; those that redistribute confiscated resources have much less compelling reasons to adopt change.

The issue of whether society in general has the obligation of providing medical care to those without the resources to provide their own is distinct from the question of whether individual practitioners have an obligation to treat those who are unable to compensate them. The concept of medicine and other healing arts as noble professions naturally assumes such an obligation, but its existence and observance are by no means certain. There are physicians and other practitioners who can practice their craft enthusiastically while purposely avoiding the destitute and indigent. If there is an obligation it does not arise from some need of the provider. The indigent likewise have no practical appeal to some overriding universal law that compels physicians to treat them without compensation. If medical ethics embraces an obligation of physicians to treat some patients regardless of compensation, such an obligation arises not from a universal principle, but from the nature of medicine and the character of those who practice it.

The philosophical analysis of obligations such as that considered here classically inquired into the nature of duty and fundamental questions of morally good and bad behavior. These inquiries tended to regress back in search of a source of the subject duty, in an attempt to identify a universal imperative that is binding upon individuals. This imperative would govern whether people agree to it or not, and regardless of whether there is a temporal authority to enforce its observance. It is rather easy, yet far from convincing, to assert that physicians should provide care to the indigent because it is required by the natural law of Aquinas or the categorical imperative of Kant. The practical issue however is not why physicians must treat the poor, but rather whether why they should.

The idea that healthcare providers should make their services available to those unable to pay for them does not derive from a stern universal authority that imposes its dictates on the willing and unwilling alike. The impetus for such selfless actions comes not so much from objective commands of a universal morality as from more subjective dispositions to charity and altruism. Medicine is a noble profession, not because it is forced to be by external authority, but because those who practice it provide that quality from their own character. Medicine did not arise as a human endeavor because wealthy people got sick; it did so because human reason and ingenuity provided a means of allowing individual people to live meaningful lives despite being subject to illness and injury. Experience and reason demonstrate that the purposes for which healers practice their arts are best served when care is motivated by the notion that every human life is worthy of those attentions that we consider virtues.

It is natural to respect and admire people for their charitable acts and commend them for their generosity. Life, quite simply, is better for everyone if it includes at least some people who perform selfless acts for the benefit of others. The development of medicine as a worthwhile human institution required the participation of people who pursued their own happiness by observing what they perceived as their moral obligations. Medicine is a worthwhile undertaking for patients, practitioners and society as a whole, and those who practice it cannot fully realize the rewards of it if they limit its benefits to those who can trade material wealth.

Doctors should provide at least some charity care because undertaking to relieve the suffering caused by illness and injury is a worthwhile undertaking in itself, and to those who truly appreciate the power of medicine to help people lead meaningful lives, it is a very elegant way to experience the fulfillment of a humanitarian undertaking.

The ethical tradition of modern medicine arises from a few simple realities, e.g. that the practice of medicine can be used for both good and bad purposes, that the effective practice of medicine requires observance of practical guidelines to enable effective care and avoid exploitation of the vulnerable, and recognition of some motives besides material gain. The ethics of modern medicine must also account for the competing interests that affect medical decisions such as the interests of society, and the moral obligations of the practitioner. These considerations form the basis of modern medical ethics and account for such various principles as physicians should safeguard patient confidences, not have romantic relationships with their patients nor refuse to treat a patient in need because that patient is indigent. They are also the basis for proscriptions against euthanasia and nonconsensual human experimentation.

The ethics of healthcare have become more complex because the production and delivery of healthcare services has become more complex. Physicians and other providers find that, in order to ensure that the modern system of healthcare remains viable, they must sometimes side with interests other than those of individual patients. Examples are found where physicians seek to have certain services or procedures reimbursed by payers that prospectively exclude them, or to have their patients given preference in systems that are designed to equitably manage insufficient resources, such as organ transplants. The former scenario undercuts the actuarial function that insurers must perform in deciding rates and estimating risk; the latter invites corruption into an undertaking that relies upon honorable motives and a sense that no person is ordinary. Physicians must do what is right for their patients, but they sometimes must also defer to the interests of society, as well as to those of the institutions that make the complex undertakings of modern healthcare possible.

6

THE BUSINESS OF MEDICINE

Medicine and the healing arts tend to become vocations and professions for their practitioners. This naturally creates a healthcare industry, and this in turn requires everyone involved in healthcare to accommodate the practical necessities of business. Business considerations are inevitable in medicine for several reasons, such as the fact that the scientific and technological bases of modern medicine are complex and expensive. A patient may be unable to anticipate or pay individually for the healthcare services that he requires, making risk-sharing arrangements through insurance risk pools a prudent strategy. The infrastructure, research, technology, facilities, personnel, training and support services required to provide modern medical care may require vast resources which must be accumulated, managed and distributed to multiple entities over periods of years or decades. These complexities beget other complexities such as regulatory compliance, amortization schedules, risk management and other legal concerns, and involve considerations such as whether a particular diagnostic or therapeutic technology is worth the investment. The cost and complexity of modern medicine by themselves require consideration and attention to matters of business.

Business concerns also arise in modern medicine because advancing the art and science of medicine involves risk, and evaluation and acceptance of risk is an inherently business-like activity. Without risk there can be no progress. In order to explore and develop novel technologies for use in the practice of medicine, it is necessary for someone to take the financial and career risk that those technologies will not succeed. In order for new treatments to be proven safe and effective it is necessary for people to subject themselves to the risks of adverse effects and the possibility that the treatment being studied will be ineffective. Even in the case of established therapies, it is necessary for the practitioner to discuss the risks and benefits of a particular course of treatment, and often to proceed against a risk of catastrophic outcome, such as death or permanent disability. Practitioners must occasionally assume risks to their own health, such as contracting a communicable disease from a patient under their care, as well as abide other professional risks, such as that of being sued for malpractice or otherwise being blamed for an undesirable outcome. Other risks are less obvious. It is impossible for an individual practitioner to become an expert in all facets of his or her practice, or to personally verify every item of clinical information regarding a patient. Practitioners must trust and rely on colleagues and other healthcare professionals to provide much of the data and interpretations necessary to patient care, but because this reliance does not transfer responsibility for the patient's care, those practitioners necessarily assume some risk that the information supplied by others will be in error.

The expense of modern medicine creates a risk to the material assets of the patient, and in some circumstances to the financial well being of the practitioners and facilities that undertake to provide care. The practice of medicine and the healing arts, like most worthwhile human activities, is fraught with risk. Success in the treatment of individual patients, as well as the progress of the art and science of medicine, requires not the mindless avoidance of risk, but the rational and unavoidable accommodation of it. Much of this accommodation, particularly that related to the financial realities of modern medicine, requires the tools and institutions of sound business practice.

The element of risk that most directly applies business concerns to the practice of medicine is that which pertains to financing the healthcare system and paying for care. Risk in this regard is an item of commerce, and businesses are involved in buying and selling the risk associated with healthcare ventures, as well as with the potentially ruinous occasion of severe illness or injury. The most familiar of these arrangements is health insurance, by which individuals contract with each other through an insurance company, and pay money to protect their assets from potentially ruinous healthcare expenses. A by-product of these arrangements is that the person who is the beneficiary of such an arrangement acquires a degree of access to medical services that might otherwise be limited if personal assets were insufficient to pay for them.

People often assume risks because they expect to be compensated for doing so. Individuals and corporations who put assets at risk to finance medical research, hospitals and other healthcare facilities, and expensive technologies make these investments with the expectation that assuming the risk of financial loss will be offset by the potential of eventual profit. Even non-profit and charitable institutions that pay for healthcare assets and services do so with the expectation that the benefit to their interests will outweigh the risk.

Business concerns enter medicine, not solely because modern healthcare requires them, but also because healthcare presents opportunities for businessmen and women to profit from it. As has been observed previously, one of the consequences of human reason is that human beings are tool users, and the human need and desire for healthcare gives rise to opportunities that can be exploited to the benefit of individual interests. It should not be expected that all participants in modern healthcare are motivated by altruistic concerns, and it is in fact quite likely that directed self-interest is responsible for much of the pace and quantity of progress in modern medicine. Healthcare services are valued by virtually all societies, and this value makes the healthcare industry amenable to exploitation for individual financial gain, and the incentive of such gain promotes improvements in efficiency and innovation.

Although considerations of risk, complexity, and self-interest provide for business participation in healthcare, the most prominent role of business in modern medicine arises from the enormous necessity of financing the healthcare system. Of all the characteristics of modern medicine apparent to the average person, one of the most obvious is that it is very expensive.

There is no single reason why modern healthcare is so expensive. Many factors contribute to this result, including the fact that the individual nature of diagnosis and therapy makes it labor-intensive. The potential harms that healthcare can cause create the necessity of cost-raising regulation to promote safe, effective care and discourage quacks and con artists. Heavy reliance on technology requires considerable amounts of research and development. These costs are unavoidable in any reasonably advanced healthcare system, but modern Western medicine, particularly that represented by that of the United States in the twenty first century entails additional, more elective costs that significantly add to its expense.

It is tempting for the average patient to assume that the expense of modern healthcare arises from fraud, waste, and the greed of healthcare industry robber barons. Healthcare professionals might assume that extraordinary expense arises because of the irresponsibility of spoiled patients, churlish doctors and meddling bureaucrats. Still others may blame tort lawyers, pharmaceutical companies, unions, demagogues, and various undefined predators. What each of these assumptions has in common is a questionable motive on the part of someone; however, it is quite likely that the extraordinary cost of American healthcare is, at least in part, a result of more benign factors and expectations. Modern healthcare is expensive because it accommodates:

1.) Performance. There is a reason why a Ferrari costs twenty times more than a Nissan Sentra, and it is not because the Ferrari goes twenty times faster or farther. Marginal increments in high performance systems cost considerably more than proportional improvements in less ambitious systems. Excellence costs disproportionately more than adequacy, and Americans want and have been willing to pay for, excellence.

2.) Access. If a patient needs a knee replaced in a fair sized American city, she can go to the local medical center, or to a specialty hospital or surgical center. These options allow patients to schedule their procedures within a reasonable time, and not subject to operative room availability that can be pre-empted by acute appendicitis, multi-trauma car accidents, dissecting aortas, or perforated bowels. Access is not only good to have in an emergency, but also provides convenience, and as is the case with 24 hour merchants, convenience is expensive. This ready access requires a certain amount of redundancy and redundancy costs money.

3.) Uncertainty. Assume a patient experiences chest pain and goes to the local hospital emergency department. A skilled practitioner can take a low technology history and physical and tell with ~85% certainty that the patient is not having a heart attack, and that he thinks the cause is esophageal spasm, or anxiety. The 15% uncertainty is unnerving, so the patient is willing to pay for cardiac enzymes that can tell with 95% certainty that the discomfort is not due to a heart attack. But the heart is important and so the patient gets admitted to an observation unit with telemetry monitoring, and because something caused the pain, receives a nuclear medicine study the next day. The ready availability of the nuclear medicine study also costs money for the same reason mentioned above. There is still uncertainty as to what caused the patient to come to the emergency room, and those involved wish to find out. The patient and physician are uncomfortable with uncertainty in such matters. The physician orders a specialized CT scan and if this doesn't answer the question the patient undergoes a swallowing study. The end result after all of these interventions and expense is the same as if the evaluation had stopped at the low-technology history and physical. If a patient is having headaches, reassurance that they are due to tension and not a tumor or an aneurysm may be a higher priority than the cost of obtaining it.

4.) Choice. A patient who is given a diagnosis of cancer might have several treatment options, the cheapest of which is disfiguring, or disabling surgery. The patient might also have the option of one the newer radiation techniques, chemotherapy protocols, highly specialized reconstruction procedures, or some highly advanced monoclonal antibody therapy. Maintaining these options and the expertise to use them costs money; money that culturally disposed societies, such as that in the United States, have been willing to spend in the private insurance market, or demand from public payers.

5.) Autonomy. There is no one other than the patient who can tell us how important the last month of his life is to him. There is no reliable way of telling that the three months he spends at home with his daughter is less meaningful than the three months that a motorcycle crash victim spends in inpatient and outpatient rehabilitation. The lifestyle and healthcare choices of individual people are matters of liberty and individual dignity, not actuarial variables to be guessed at by remote bureaucrats. It is much cheaper for treatment decisions to be made by accountants; it is much more meaningful for these same decisions to be made by unique and irreplaceable people.

6.) Fantasy. We all engage in illusions that are comforting or that provide emotional reassurance, even if we know these illusions are contrary to reality. We assume that the natural condition of mankind is to die of old age, at home surrounded by loved ones. We want to think that our doctors will succeed in whatever therapeutic interventions they try, regardless of what reason tells us, and if the outcome is less than expected, a jury may be asked to provide recourse. We want to pretend that the 87 year old who just had a massive stroke will get back on her feet "because she's always been active," as soon as she is able to eat. As a consequence we are willing to spend significant money for what may be a one-in-a-hundred shot. We do this, not because we are greedy or stupid, but because we look at our loved ones a certain way. It may be, in the case of healthcare, that these are futile expenditures, but the underlying presumption, that human life is never an ordinary thing, permeates what we do and what we value as a society. The money we spend on fantastic healthcare ambitions is often a consequence of our values.

7.) Responsiveness. Ambulances and emergency rooms respond to everyone who has a medical emergency based only on the fact that the patient is a human being. It requires infrastructure to ensure 24-hour coverage, aerial transport if necessary, and tertiary care centers when needed. Americans have not only been willing to pay for these services, but have demanded them.

8.) Distorted markets. The third-party payer system insulates the patient from the true expenses of the services they receive, and mitigates the financial disincentives that discourage services that have little or no benefit.

9.) Ancillary interests. Healthcare services are consumed for reasons other than the diagnosis and treatment of illness and injury. Common examples of such scenarios are a physician ordering tests to limit liability exposure, or a patient demanding a CT scan to rule out a condition she just heard about on daytime television, without clinical suspicion of disease. Patients are encouraged to request therapies on the thinnest indications through direct marketing by pharmaceutical and medical device manufacturers. Hospitals have an incentive to encourage use of expensive imaging devices in order to recoup their investments. Expensive healthcare services remain expensive even when their use is not primarily to benefit the patient.

The fact that healthcare, particularly modern American healthcare, is so expensive is not due to an isolated characteristic of its delivery. The expense of healthcare is largely a by-product of cultural values. The huge marginal costs of healthcare expenditures goes to providing a relatively small amount of high-performance services. The Pareto principle suggests that 80% of healthcare services result from 20% of the expenditures, and conversely, 20% of the high-end services consume 80% of the costs. The ratios are obviously somewhat arbitrary, but do serve to illustrate the fact that a disproportionate amount of healthcare resources are consumed in intensive care units, tertiary care facilities in the last weeks of life, and in interventions with low likelihood of clinical success. "Basic" healthcare, meaning that which is required by people who are not very sick, is relatively cheap, but Americans have come to expect (and apparently are willing to pay for) much more than the basics.

Because modern healthcare is so expensive, those involved with the business of medicine are engaged in two ongoing endeavors: trying to make medicine less expensive and figuring out how to pay for it. There are many rational strategies for reducing the cost of healthcare, however some approaches sound much better in theory than they prove to be in practice. One way to make healthcare less expensive is to eliminate or reduce the very high cost items that it contains. Such an approach inevitably leads to denying high cost care to patients who seek it, and thus rationing is a final common pathway of many healthcare reform efforts.

Rationing is an effective method of limiting healthcare expenses by simply limiting healthcare. It is an effective brute force economic method of trading off the cost of healthcare against the presumed benefits that such care provides. The unavoidable trading-off character is the element of rationing that provides the greatest potential for conflict with more established values. The simplest form of rationing is the creation of rules by which patients are denied care as a result of defined, inflexible criteria. These criteria may apply to the type of care being sought, the patient seeking it, the location of the patient, or a combination of such factors. Cost cutting by this method causes unease, because there is something inherently dystopian about refusing joint replacement surgery to an octogenarian, simply because she is an octogenarian, or terminating dialysis in a thriving patient because he has used up his allotment. Rationing in this manner conjures up references to death panels, eugenics and heartless bureaucracies.

Accommodating such ideas in modern societies requires an uncomfortable adjustment in the way people view their relationships with each other, their healthcare providers and their society. Because of this, reformers often propose other, less overt forms of rationing. With reference to the expense-driving factors mentioned above, a degree of rationing could be achieved by limiting the choice of facilities available to patients, forcing them to accept care in only the lowest cost ones. Expensive air ambulance costs can be curtailed by eliminating some air ambulance services, at the risk that some patients will experience worse outcomes as a result. This approach to rationing makes certain services available in theory but limits access to them in practice.

Another form of rationing is suggested by the excess expense of very high acuity interventions. Keeping severely ill and debilitated patients alive, much less curing them, with extraordinary interventions is obviously much more expensive than is limiting therapy to less sophisticated treatments. Furthermore, it can be assumed that the population of patients who require the advanced therapies is much smaller than that population that does not. It is an obvious but useful axiom that it costs less to care for people who are relatively healthy than it does to care for those who are very sick. This is the reason why the healthcare systems of less developed countries appear more cost-efficient than more developed ones. Those that are highly developed are more willing to expend significant resources on a relatively small population that is likely to have a poor outcome regardless of the intervention, whereas the less aggressive system achieves the approximately same outcome at no additional cost.

The vast majority of medical problems can be treated with relatively cost effective interventions. The addition of very expensive, high tech care adds disproportionate costs in a population that is relatively small, and where the risk of therapeutic failure is greater. As a matter of unsophisticated observation, a certain amount of medical problems for which people seek care are transient conditions that will resolve without any intervention by the healthcare system. Of those that require intervention, a certain percentage will respond adequately to the care of non-specialist, or even non-physician providers, who can direct the patient to standard therapies without sophisticated diagnostic studies. Of those patients and their conditions remaining, some will require the services of highly trained specialists, and successful therapy will involve very advanced and expensive care. Basic healthcare systems tend to direct patients toward less sophisticated therapies, but in very advanced and technology-dependent healthcare systems, patients tend to be shunted toward the more advanced interventions. This phenomenon is the result of risk aversion, commercial interests, and patient expectations. A subtle form of rationing would limit patient's access to more advanced services until after they have failed more basic care.

An effective method of rationing is to force patients to wait for care in queues. This is accomplished by reducing the amount of redundancy that otherwise is available to limit wait-times, and follows the premise that some people who are forced to wait long periods for care eventually will not get it at all. Queues introduce an element of inconvenience that self-selects the more legitimate medical complaints, and leads those less urgent to conclude that it is not worth the trouble. It also occasionally forces patients to wait for services beyond the point that they will do any good. As with other forms of rationing, the use of protracted wait times inevitably leads to an increase in undesirable outcomes and raises questions of whether that is acceptable to current values. All forms of enforced cost cutting involve some manner of rationing, and consequently some form of denial. The result is sometimes undesirable consequences that might otherwise be avoided.

Another approach to limiting healthcare costs is to increase the efficiency of healthcare delivery. Efficiency is simply the amount of something desirable that is produced per unit of resource; e.g. miles per gallon, customers per hour, or bushels per acre. With regard to the financing of healthcare, the pertinent ratio is the value of care per unit cost. This type of efficiency is often referred to as "cost effectiveness." All other things being equal, cost effective medicine is preferable to that which is not. The development of modern medicine has been a triumph of human progress, and progress requires efficiency. All progress is really just an improvement of the efficiency of something, and efficient organisms survive at the expense of the inefficient ones.

Measuring the efficiency of healthcare is not always straightforward, because the value of care is difficult to determine. The value of some types of care, such as the attention of a nurse or the intangible experience of an accomplished physician is difficult to measure. Different patients may perceive similar outcomes differently and there may be variations in the quality of care that are important to patients, but that are not considered in determining cost effectiveness. For example, two patients may be treated for similar lung infections and ultimately experience the same outcome, but one patient uses a therapy that must be taken more frequently and is associated with nausea or itching. Even thought the amount of care may appear similar, one course of therapy may have characteristics that make it much more desirable than the other, and thus of greater value to the patient. Similar outcomes do not translate into similar value, and considering value introduces a measure of subjectivity that makes cost effectiveness itself something of a subjective determination.

In order to make calculation of cost effectiveness more uniform and comparable, healthcare managers seek the most objective measures upon which to base their analysis. This process is limited, however, by the fact that the purposes and goals of healthcare have always been personal and subjective. Cost effectiveness is often discussed in terms of easily measured variables, such as the years of life saved per unit of cost, or the years of functional life, etc. In trying to make the metrics more exact, healthcare economists invariably begin to consider parameters that are subjective and difficult to quantify, such as the number of quality years of life. Amputating an infected limb or performing a radical mastectomy cannot be directly compared with less disfiguring alternatives because it is difficult to appraise disfigurement, or to quantify the importance that a patient will attach to the adverse consequences of a particular therapy.

The usefulness of cost effectiveness is sometimes limited because different ways of calculating it produce conflicting results. An example of such a situation is the treatment of aspiration pneumonia, a condition that results when contents of the mouth are inhaled into the lungs. Patients at high risk of aspiration include those suffering strokes or other neuromuscular diseases. The incidence increases with age, and it also affects patients using recreational drugs or therapies that depress the level of consciousness. A simple question would seem to be "is it cost effective to treat aspiration pneumonia?" The answer is not straightforward. Even though the treatment tends to be simple and relatively inexpensive, consisting of antibiotics and supportive care, the financial consequences of such treatment varies from one patient to another. Curing a single episode of aspiration pneumonia does not involve extraordinary expense, and if the patient is otherwise healthy, and the cause of the aspiration transient, a good outcome involves relatively little cost. However if the condition that predisposed the patient to episode is chronic or degenerative, successful treatment may simply be a prelude to expensive and increasingly ineffective care, with little meaningful difference to the patient.

Even though the concept of cost effectiveness is inherently limited by the subjective value of healthcare, it does have a role in determining how interventions and procedures compare with each other based on objective criteria, and independent of the individual preferences of particular patients. It is useful in allocating limited resources, and determining which interventions are best and least suited to those aims.

Technology has made significant contributions to the cost effectiveness of medicine. Advanced diagnostic methods can detect certain diseases at earlier, more easily treated stages. Robotic and fiber optic techniques make surgery less invasive and thus reduce recovery times and associated complications. Other technologies, such as electronic health records and computer-based evaluations that allow physicians to evaluate patient data and prescribe therapies without physical proximity to the patient, make medical practice less cumbersome. These innovations, like many advanced technologies, become cheaper the more they are used, developed and refined. This is one of the great conundrums facing healthcare policy makers. Technology costs money but can also produce greater efficiency. Progress is expensive, but pays off in the long run.

Because efficiency is one of the goals of medical progress, it would seem that the prospects for achieving it are unlimited. In practice however, the value of healthcare derives as much from the personal interactions as it does from the use of medical technology. There is a limit to the extent that technology can influence the nurse-to-patient ratio in an intensive care unit, or to how many minutes of physician consultation time it can replace. Healthcare is a highly labor-intensive undertaking, much of the benefit of which derives from the fact that it is labor-intensive. One observation, attributed to Daniel Patrick Moynihan, but which may have originated with others, is that there is a practical limit to the efficiency of systems that require close personal interactions. Mr. Moynihan was speaking specifically about the education system, but the observation is equally valid for healthcare. Much of the value and effect of healthcare derives from the relationships between patients and providers. The human element of modern healthcare is unlikely to be replaced by technology, or made more efficient by systemic tinkering. In some ways the relentless pursuit of efficiency can appear dehumanizing, and when this perception invades the relationships between patients and providers, it makes the whole effort somewhat moot.

Another factor limiting the achievable efficiency of the healthcare system is government regulation. Useful oversight entails significant amounts of data collection, review, and compliance costs. All of these divert money from direct healthcare services. Moreover, regulations often must balance competing interests, such as the risk and efficacy of particular treatments, privacy concerns and availability of patient data, and ease of access and quality of care provided by various facilities. The more interests that are accommodated in the healthcare system, e.g. cost-effectiveness, access, liability for adverse outcomes, shorter waiting times, availability of imaging studies, etc., the more that efficiency will decline. Accommodation of competing interests unavoidably introduces inefficiencies, and modern healthcare is replete with competing interests.

A considerable amount of thought, resources, effort and planning goes into figuring out how to finance healthcare. In practice there are three distinct payment sources that have particular benefits and drawbacks in financing a complex healthcare system. The first is the person who uses healthcare, which is the patient or someone acting for the patient's benefit. Financing healthcare solely through the individual resources of the patient has become largely impractical because of the ballooning cost of healthcare. It is common for the expenses related to a serious accident or injury to equal years of a person's annual income. It is possible for patients with certain chronic conditions such as rheumatoid arthritis or Crohn's disease to pay more for their monthly medications than they do for housing. It is simply impractical for the complex, integrated and highly capital-intensive healthcare system to be financed by point-of-care payments from individual patients at the time they receive care. This is true, in no small measure because many patients will not have the resources make such payments.

One obvious solution to the inability of individual people to provide for their own care is to share the risk that any of them will incur medical expenses that would prove to be financially ruinous. This is the concept behind health insurance, although as noted, it does not insure health as much as it does the assets of patients facing massive healthcare expenses. Pooling of resources creates a fund from which individual medical expenses can be paid, with the desirable consequence that providers will have more confidence that they will be compensated for the services they provide. This has the effect of making services available to insured patients, where providers may be less willing to bear the risk that an uninsured patient's assets will leave a shortfall. There are other benefits to the insurance model. The risk of disease and injury, as well as the costs of treating them are items that can be assessed and managed. Doing so requires a great deal of data and sophisticated analysis tools that are beyond the abilities of a typical individual. Insurers have an incentive to identify and encourage risk-reducing strategies, as well as evaluate the benefit and cost effectiveness of various diagnostic and therapeutic interventions.

Private financing of healthcare is inherently compatible with market regulation of costs. Market mechanisms introduce competition, and competition is a very effective optimizing mechanism. Competition selects out the most efficient market participants and in markets, as in nature, the more efficient survive at the expense of the less efficient.

The private financing of healthcare services, either directly from individual patients or through privately contracted insurance arrangements, has an additional advantage. The purposes for which people seek treatment for illness and injury are unavoidably concerned with individual values. When patients either pay for their own care or contract with others of similar ideals they can seek out those services most consistent with their own views and beliefs. The private financing of healthcare, in theory, allows a measure of autonomy that is lost when patients must abide by the preferences of those who pay the bills.

A theoretical benefit of insurers is that, conceptually, they are disinterested intermediaries; they merely facilitate the process by which individuals contract with each other for the purpose of spreading and managing risk. In practice, however, the insurer is more than just a risk sharing collective. It is a business enterprise with its own interests that may or may not always be consistent with that of its insureds. The services that insurance companies provide are valuable and wherever there is value there is a potential for profit. Those who seek to profit from insurance of medical risk have interests that are inherently different from, and not infrequently in conflict with, those of individual patients. Situations may arise when certain therapies are very expensive, but might still provide benefits over less costly alternatives. In such cases, the interest of the insured in having access to those therapies will conflict with the insurance company's shareholders' interest in a return on their investments.

The pure market-based private insurance model has other drawbacks as well. The voluntary nature of individuals contracting with each other to share risks makes it possible to exclude those who might represent an excessive burden on the finances of such an arrangement. The maxim that it is cheaper to care for people who are less sick than it is to care for those who are very sick serves to identify a population that would naturally be excluded from the benefits of a market based insurance model for financing healthcare. This may conflict with other concepts of the relationship between members in a society and the view of healthcare as something more than a commercial enterprise. While private arrangements involving patients, providers, investors and insurance companies, in various combinations, can make positive contributions to the financing of healthcare, their limitations preclude them from being universally applicable.

The profit motive provides a very strong incentive to nearly all forms of progress. Injecting profit into every endeavor, however, often jeopardizes aspects of those endeavors that are motivated by more humanitarian concerns. Healthcare, being a quintessential human endeavor and often attending circumstances of profound pathos and empathy, quite naturally stimulates altruism in many people. Charity has always been an inherent part of healthcare, fulfilling vital roles when neither profit motives nor government institutions were sufficient to the task. The threat of exploitation when profit motives are present, such as the selling of organs for transplant and political concerns that burden government decision making, require altruistic motives for certain types of care to be culturally acceptable and ethically permissible. Charitable organizations are essential to such situations. In addition, some people regard the humanitarian and sacrificial aspects of charity as essential to the process of healing, such as those who view faith-based interventions as essential to meaningful healthcare services.

Charitable institutions have existed and thrived for thousands of years. Charity itself has survived and come to be revered as a virtue because it is useful to those institutions that have embraced it. Charitable sentiments are part of many religious traditions, and are sometimes even regarded as ethical obligations. Charity has beneficial effects on the relationships between people who live among each other despite differences in circumstances and fortunes. Charitable communities in general are more stable and more cohesive than those that are less giving. Generosity is a not only a trait of admirable character, it is a necessary virtue among people that are interdependent. The perception that people donate resources to be devoted to the care and comfort of others, without tangible recompense to the giver, creates the sense that providing healthcare is worthwhile simply because it is the right thing to do.

Charitable organizations have founded and sustained entire hospital systems. They were sometimes the only institutions capable of or willing to provide healthcare in certain locations and to certain populations. They have underwritten significant amounts of medical research, and provided care to people who otherwise could afford none. Despite this, there is skepticism that charitable processes are reliable enough to sustain substantial parts of modern healthcare systems. Charitable contributions are always somewhat sensitive to underlying economic conditions, and modern life provides no shortage of worthy causes besides healthcare. Charity based healthcare also suffers from something of an image problem because of a popular sentiment that there is something demeaning or undignified in relying on the beneficence of strangers. Furthermore, charitable organizations typically reflect a discrete set of values that may or may not be consistent with the values of those who seek care. This is a drawback of government financed healthcare as well, and considering how intimately individual values are intertwined with the purposes of healthcare, it is not an insignificant consideration. Charitable financing of healthcare services would seem to be a necessary, but not sufficient, part of modern medicine.

Because individually financed healthcare, including that achieved through risk sharing insurance arrangements, may leave impoverished patients without access to care, and exclusive reliance on charitable financing may be unreliable or provoke clashes of incompatible values, people understandably look to government to remedy these drawbacks.

Government involvement in healthcare financing is attractive because governments are perceived as having certain powers that may useful to the enterprise, specifically, a large and elastic source of funds, and the ability to enforce compliance with its rules and regulations through the use of force. Government involvement also leaves the impression that healthcare services are regarded as a societal obligation, and that its ability to fulfill that obligation is a measure of progress and justice.

There is a level of confidence that attaches to government-financed healthcare that arises from an assumption that the government will make good on public obligations. Insurers may become insolvent, and charities can experience shortfalls that cannot be remedied by other means, but beneficiaries of a publicly funded payer can be reassured by the government's ability to borrow money, or tax needed funds from the resources of private citizens when necessary.

The ability of governments to mandate and proscribe theoretically eliminates much of the uncertainty that accompanies complex transactions. Deficiencies that arise from inability to stay competitive with other healthcare system participants can be addressed, at least superficially, by fiat. An imbalance in the availability of certain therapies that may be occasioned by the efficiency of markets can be countered by statute or regulation. Governmentally enforced compliance can at least attempt to make some services available to people who otherwise would have none, and ensure that those services that are provided do not stray too far from accepted cultural values and political interests. Whether this attribute of government-financed healthcare is a good thing or a bad thing depends on the ultimate consequences of such compulsion.

Limiting the pitfalls of market-based financing systems by using the coercive power of the state sounds better in theory than it works in practice. Despite the attempt to counter undesirable effects of market driven healthcare services, the forces that create those effects do not go away simply because the government enacts regulations that are contrary to them. Attempts to limit the cost of services quite naturally limit the supply of them. Programs that seek to expand access to certain types of healthcare have unpredictable effects on demand for those services, or upon the actual cost. Once a government agency promulgates a rule or regulation, even with the most earnest and benevolent of motives, rational people will exploit those regulations in ways not always anticipated by those that draft them. In 1966, after enactment of Medicare, the Congressional Ways and Means Committee estimated that the program would cost an inflation-adjusted 12 billion dollars in 1990; the actual cost was 107 billion dollars. Unpleasant realities that differ wildly from earnest predictions are not the result of venal or incompetent policy makers. Unexpected and undesirable results are often due to the unpredictability of the mechanisms used to achieve a stated goal. This is especially so when the government resorts to mandates and prohibitions to accomplish some narrow policy objective, but which stimulates an unwanted response in the population that is affected. The intrusion of unintended consequences is invited by policies that must accommodate too many interests that are constrained by political concerns, and that default to the most convenient, rather than the most effective, remedies for latent shortcomings.

Government involvement in healthcare introduces a number of limitations into the delivery of services. Government action is almost always colored by political concerns, and while politics is an inherent part of any societal institution, it is not generally a fundamental concern of a particular patient seeking treatment for a particular condition. The values that permeate delivery of medical services in a government-financed model may or may not be consistent with the values of the patients and providers that use and provide those services. The political and bureaucratic processes that lead to regulations and generalized policies would not be expected to produce the same economic outcomes that market based mechanisms provide, nor reflect the varying interests and values that are part of the individual interactions between patients and providers. A system that is dominated by the government lacks the optimizing mechanism of competition, and the ability to tax and compel, regulate and prohibit is an inadequate substitute.

Government planners are often unable to predict the shifting demands and expectations that people have of the healthcare system, and responses to such demands are dampened by bureaucratic inertia, risk aversion and corruption.

There is no perfect model for financing healthcare services in an advanced society. This is so because of the variety of values, which sometimes conflict with each other, the plethora of competing interests that are disposed to exploit the weaknesses in any funding mechanism, and the lack of a universal method to address mismatches between healthcare demand and healthcare resources. The challenge is to find the right balance of elements from various models; the correct proportions that harmonize the several interests, values and economic realities. This balance is always changing, however, because the interests, values and realties are not static, and certainly the practice of the healing arts itself is always changing.

The ability to provide and pay for healthcare services is limited by practical realities. The demand for such services is not determined merely by objective considerations of health and disease, but also by psychological, cultural and economic factors. The demand is further affected by distortions in market behavior that occur when the parties consuming particular services are not the ones that directly pay for them. The supply of healthcare services, in contrast, is subject to hard realities that are immune to emotional appeals and the often-neglected shortcomings of good intentions. In a very practical way, healthcare is a limited resource that requires wise stewardship and frequently difficult choices. Because of this, any system for paying for healthcare in a civilized and humane society must account for such abstract but necessary considerations of fairness and justice.

Fairness is essential to the survival of any system that involves complex transactions and interactions among people. Fairness as a quality has an almost universal appeal, and is almost instinctively regarded as desirable, especially in matters involving competition among disparate interests, or when limited resources are to be distributed. The persuasive power of appeals to fairness is such that the term is sometimes misapplied to other considerations such as mercy or compassion. In reality, mercy and compassion are often invoked to negate the harsh consequences of systems that are otherwise fair. Almost by definition, fairness is cold-blooded, and often heartless. A fair system should not favor the emotionally appealing any more than it should the economically powerful or politically connected. Confusion over this point arises because fairness is often assumed to result in desirable outcomes.

Fairness is not a characteristic of a particular result; rather it is an attribute of the process that leads to the result. Nearly all competitive athletic contests have winners and losers; outcomes with a demonstrably unequal quality. If a basketball team loses a game to a more talented and experienced opponent the outcome most certainly is not equal, but if the game was played according to the rules with impartial officials, the losing side has no grounds for appealing the unequal result as unfair. Likewise if two parties agree to determine ownership of a large sum of money by flipping a coin, the process will be fair, even if the outcome provides a windfall to one and leaves the other with nothing. If a coin is flipped to determine which of two children receives an organ transplant the process is no less fair even though the outcome for one is lamentable. Fairness implies that the process under consideration was free of improper influence, and was not tainted by extraneous considerations that would favor one outcome over another. Often times, there can be no more fair process than leaving outcomes to fate or chance, although the resulting outcomes may seem wanton or even cruel. Avoiding such results by mandating particular outcomes makes the perceived fairness of the process meaningless.

Fairness is very desirable in some situations and less so in others. Processes that yield the optimizing effect of competition work best when those processes are fair. Fair processes tend to mitigate resentments that might otherwise attend unavoidably unequal outcomes. Fairness finds particular application in matters of health and illness because those matters are quite often the result of, if not bad luck, then blind chance. The very human observation of who gets sick or injured, who gets better and who does not, almost instinctively leads to the conclusion that matters of health, disease and injury are not fair.

Fair processes are those that are free of extraneous biases, including those that favor outcomes that might be regarded as more compassionate, or more equal, or perhaps simply more emotionally satisfying. Fairness is not an end in itself, but a quality that protects complex interactions and exchanges between people from the deterioration of corruption. Fair processes often produce results that conflict with other interests, and for this reason fairness, even when desirable, may be an insufficient basis upon which to judge the allocation of healthcare resources. In such cases, the outcomes may be scrutinized, not to determine if the processes that produced them are fair, but whether the outcomes themselves are just.

Justice is another quality that is essential to the interactions between people in a society. In its most elemental form, justice is the appropriateness of the consequences of specific choices and actions. The criminal law seeks to apply appropriate sanctions for socially harmful behavior; civil law attempts to balance the benefits and burdens of the choices and conduct of individual persons in their interactions with others, through enforcement of contracts, providing compensation for negligence or intentional harm, and providing recourse for violation of individual rights. Justice is indispensable to all societies that are advanced to any degree. Because it is concerned with the relationship between behavior and consequences, it naturally encourages beneficial conduct and discourages that which is harmful. Since justice is desirable when individuals interact with each other and indispensable when they must live peacefully among each other, it would seem to be a necessary attribute of any system of financing healthcare for any appreciable number of people. This principle is much easier to conceive in theory than apply in practice however.

The assertion that a particular person should receive a particular healthcare service, by itself, provides no insight into the grounds upon which it is made. It is not obvious that the person should receive care for an injury or illness because of a "social contract" obligation to provide such care, because providing such care is compassionate and dictated by civilized notions of humane behavior, because the person is entitled to treatment because the concept of justice gives him a claim on the healthcare resources of the society of which he is a part, or perhaps a little of each. This is a practical problem for policy makers and philosophers alike, since attributing access to some services to notions of compassion and others to notions of justice is inconsistent with notions of either compassion or justice. A process that seeks to determine who is worthy of compassion and who is not, itself lacks compassion. Similarly explaining how justice establishes a basis for one person's heart bypass, but not another's is likely to lead to a contradiction. Furthermore, the abstract world where justice is omnipotent does not translate readily into more concrete realities. It is difficult, if not impossible, to argue that considerations of justice explain why one child gets a heart transplant and another does not, or why a resident of a rural community will not receive the same treatment for his stroke as a will a similarly afflicted resident of a large city. Justice cannot explain why a nonagenarian with advanced dementia receives dialysis in an overcrowded outpatient center while a young immigrant must rely on weekly visits to an emergency room under an assumed name to receive the same treatment. Justice, by itself, gives little recourse to anyone trying to understand the disparate attention given to those suffering from cancer and those afflicted with schizophrenia.

These observations are not meant to imply that considerations of societal obligation, compassion, justice, or any other rationale that serves as a basis for allocating often-limited healthcare resources are invalid. Rather, they illustrate that when competing interests and practical limitations affect provision of healthcare services, it is not a single abstract virtue or criterion that controls. As in many areas of life, it is culture, competing interests, communal values, and sometimes luck that determine the outcome.

7

THE MODERN PRACTICE OF MEDICINE

When people are afflicted with an injury or illness, they seek out the services of a healthcare provider, with the expectation that the professional expertise of that provider will produce a remedy for their complaint. While knowledge and technical skill are essential to the successful practice of medicine, what distinguishes the profession of medicine from a healthcare trade is the professional's proficiency in making decisions. The capacity to make decisions is essential not only to the medical profession, but to professions generally, applying to attorneys, accountants, military officers, airline pilots and mutual fund managers. Many parts of modern life require decisions to be made based on complex data, involving significant risks and appreciable uncertainty, and in subtle contexts. Mechanical application of generalized rules is insufficient in such environments and people naturally seek the judgment and insight of professionals.

Medical decision-making often requires professional expertise because the data upon which such decisions are made may be conflicting, incomplete, or inaccurate. It is not always obvious that a patient's symptoms are the direct result of a pathologic process, rather than the body's natural response to therapy. The disease processes or injuries with which patients present may not be fully understood, or may evade the usual methods of diagnosis. They may respond to conventional therapies in unpredictable and undesirable ways. Often times the only thing that is certain after the usual work-up is that the patient is ill and that there is no obvious intervention to reliably provide a cure, yet the professional is expected to do something about it anyway. People do not strictly need a physician when both the diagnosis and therapeutic interventions are obvious. People need physicians and other healthcare professionals when uncertainty, confusion, novelty and unpleasant surprises accompany the patient's complaint.

The reality of medical decision-making is that the professional must often make decisions under stressed time constraints and in less than ideal circumstances. The data that are available to the practitioner are often surrogates for the true item of interest, and the correlation between the two may be imperfect. An example of such a surrogate and its correlate is the body temperature and the presence of bacterial infection. This association creates significant temptation to prescribe antibiotics based on the presence of elevated body temperature, despite the fact that inappropriate use of antibiotics is accompanied by significant undesirable consequences. Further data, such as the white blood cell count, x-ray findings and the patient's symptoms may either confirm or refute the initial presumption of infection. These additional data are likewise imperfectly correlated with the diagnosis under consideration, and treatment decisions may come down to an educated guess or the intuition of an experienced provider.

The uncertainties of modern medical practice are not limited to those that accompany issues of diagnosis and therapy. There may be uncertainty as to the patient's goals or reason for seeking healthcare services or there may be questions as to the patient's ability and desire to adhere to burdensome therapeutic regimens. The risk of a particular treatment in a particular patient may be unknown. There may be significant psychological components to a patient's symptoms and response to intervention, as well as financial and regulatory barriers to desired courses of treatment. There may be little in a patient's presentation to help the practitioner distinguish a community acquired influenza infection that will get better on its own in a few days from a more complicated variety that will become fatal in a matter of hours. On occasion, it is not only the appropriate course of treatment that is uncertain, but the desired outcome as well.

Accommodating uncertainty is not the only challenge that confronts modern medical decision-making. Medical decisions entail risk assessment and management, consideration of competing interests, and ethical as well as practical constraints on therapeutic options. The risks involved in medical treatment range from the trivial to the lethal, and involve not only the patient's health but also the interests of other healthcare system participants.

Risk avoidance is sometimes a dominant concern in medical decision-making and is the underlying motive for what is commonly termed defensive medicine. Physicians may be motivated to order low-yield tests to minimize claims of careless practice, or prefer less beneficial therapies if they also carry a lower chance of unanticipated outcomes. Risk avoidance is a pervasive phenomenon that often operates independently of the patient's welfare, and is often simply a consequence of conflicting interests. The person seeking to avoid an undesirable risk, whether that risk is of a potential lawsuit, excessive cost or adverse outcomes prioritizes evasion of that risk above other considerations related to the patient's care.

The decision-making aspect of modern medical practice implies a certain degree of discretion on the part of the practitioner. If the practitioner has no discretion regarding the care that he or she provides, there is no room for decision-making and the healthcare provider then becomes more of a technician. Discretion is necessary in medicine for the simple reason that disease and injury have innumerable possible presentations, and the data necessary to definitively characterize them are frequently scant and insufficient. The same complaint of pain in two different patients may be due to processes that are innocuous in the one and catastrophic in the other, with no definite way to distinguish the two. Discretion is also needed where the risks of the same therapy vary between patients, such as using a blood thinner in a patient who has a history of bleeding ulcers and in a patient who does not. Discretion is necessary in situations where the practitioner must interpret conflicting clinical information, or where the patient may be reluctant to provide an accurate account of symptoms or response to treatment.

One of the reasons that discretion is inherent in the practice of medicine is that there is not a deterministic relationship between diseases and injuries, diagnostic efforts and treatments. Anyone could be a healer if the diagnosis and appropriate therapy were never in doubt. The reality of medicine however is that the practitioner is expected to make some part of the patient's life better, even if the identity of the malady is unknown or, if known, there is no available cure. The art of medicine is not so much doing the right thing when all the facts are known, as much as doing a helpful thing when the facts are unknown, or the prognosis is unalterable. This expectation further highlights the difference between professionals and technicians.

Discretion, however, may also be associated with certain pitfalls. It may serve as a cover for inattentiveness or poor judgment. Unfettered discretion makes it impossible to establish standardized diagnostic and treatment regimens for common conditions, and at least allows the possibility that treatment decisions will reflect the tastes and fashions of the provider, rather than the best practices that reason and experience can provide.

To avoid these pitfalls, various authoritative bodies have undertaken to standardize certain elements of medical practice. Expert panels and medical bureaucracies promulgate treatment guidelines, clinical pathways and treatment algorithms. The end result is often a more standardized approach to treatment of a particular conditions, as well as objective checklists to ensure that important treatment considerations are not foregone out of carelessness or haste. The tradeoff for this objective compulsiveness is that treatment decisions can end up being made by remote committees that never see the particular patient whose care they are affecting. The guidelines and algorithms that dictate specific diagnostic and treatment decisions may be based on considerations of a population of patients that may or may not include the individual patient being treated, and it is possible that what has been shown to have a statistical benefit for a large, selected group of patients will be disastrous for a particular patient.

Despite the distinguishing characteristic of medical practice as that of learned decision-making, medical practice is becoming more dependent on guidelines, protocols, flow charts, clinical pathways and checklists; a situation that is derisively referred to as "cookbook medicine." The proliferation of these decision guides is the result of multiple factors. Guidelines and protocols are perceived as a method of accumulating expertise and specialized experience into a form available to the individual practitioner. They are also a method of condensing and disseminating the most up-to-date methods of diagnosis and treatment. They also serve the same function that checklists do in aviation: objective guides to ensure that essential considerations are not overlooked. In some circumstances, these decision guides might be considered obligatory, not guidelines but mandates. Institutions may be prone to impose these formal rules and procedures on the physicians who practice there, and the motivation is not always to ensure the most appropriate care for the patient. Discretion involves some consideration of alternatives, with the unavoidable risk that the decision maker will select an inappropriate alternative. Rigid adherence to guidelines has the effect of limiting discretion, and therefore risk, and the natural history of institutions is often that they become increasingly risk averse. It is much easier to avoid accountability for a decision if one can claim that another compelled it. Discretion is often regarded as an element of fault, and guidelines, protocols and algorithms may be seen as methods of avoiding liability. This can either be good or bad, but the increasing intrusion of centralized and remote rule-making into specific medical decisions seems to be based on the assumption that discretion is not a always a good thing. Sometimes poorly drafted or reasoned guidelines are misapplied with detrimental results. In medicine, as in other areas of life, mindless guidelines are often followed mindlessly.

There is no definitive answer to whether a particular patient is better served by the informed discretion of his individual practitioner, or by the standardizing approach that relies on remote expertise. Some patients will benefit more from the former, others from the latter. In general, discretion is most useful in evaluating and interpreting clinical data, and clinical guidelines and protocols are more useful for ensuring that such data are obtained and considered. Discretion is most valuable in making individualized treatment decisions; guidelines are helpful for ensuring that appropriate treatment results from those decisions.

Medical decision-making, and thus, the professional practice of modern medicine, is heavily influenced by the methods of science and scientific reasoning. The reason that practitioners can prescribe specific therapies in particular clinical circumstances is because the scientific approach of observation and experimentation allows reasonable predictions of the outcomes of such therapies. It was certainly valid and astute observation that led medieval physicians to treat the excess urine production associated with diabetes mellitus with portions of the French lilac plant, without knowing that the guanidine contained in that plant lowered the patient's blood sugar, and therefore interrupted the process leading to large urine output. Subsequent research and investigation identified the mechanism of this effect, giving scientific validity to this manner of therapy.

Once the details of the pathology and the mechanism of the treatment are understood, it is possible to make rational predictions regarding the effect of treatment on the given condition, and this serves as an ideal to which modern medicine aspires. In reality however, much of the practice of medicine is decidedly unscientific. This is not due to casualness regarding scientific rigor, as much as it is due to the ethical and practical constraints of medical practice being incompatible with scientific methods of inquiry. It is simply not ethically possible to conduct scientifically rigorous studies that involve disfiguring "sham" surgeries, or to withhold known efficacious therapies to assess a novel treatment against an untreated control population. Good science must sometimes defer to good ethics.

Scientists sometimes try to accommodate the ethical limitations on medical research by using laboratory animals such as rats. While this strategy avoids many of the ethical constraints on human experimentation, for the simple and obvious reason that rats are not humans, this characteristic imposes limitations of its own. For example, in the 1970s experiments on laboratory rats raised concerns that the artificial sweetener saccharin was linked to bladder cancer. The Food and Drug Administration announced in 1973 that it had "presumptive evidence" that saccharin caused bladder cancer in rats. Bladder tumors were found in three of 48 rats that consumed saccharin as 7.5% of their diet. As a result, the government required that all food containing saccharin carry a warning of suspected health risks. This labeling requirement was rescinded in 2000 however, after it was discovered that differences in urinary chemistry between humans and rats likely accounted for the occurrence of cancers in the latter. Processes occurred in rat urine that produced micro-crystals that were damaging to the lining of the bladder, but these processes did not normally occur in humans. Clinical experience did not confirm the theoretical carcinogenic effect of saccharine in human beings.

Even where there are no limiting ethical concerns, the practice of medicine sometimes incorporates theories that are incomplete or misunderstood, and also adopts erroneous deductions that are mistaken for scientific conclusions. In the 1990s, it was widely accepted that hormone replacement therapy was a rational method of limiting cardiovascular disease risk in menopausal women. This premise had not only a theoretical basis, but preliminary clinical data seemed to validate it. Subsequent experience however showed that not only was the benefit overstated, but that there were accompanying risks of stroke and blood clots that undermined the prudence of routine hormone replacement therapy.

Sometimes, science validates therapeutic interventions with great fanfare, and these interventions become standard treatment for years. Those years of experience then, on closer examination, reveal that the original validation was faulty and that the intervention is not good medicine. The clinical syndrome known as sepsis that accompanies severe infections has always been associated with considerable mortality and there were few effective treatment options other than aggressive life support and treatment of the underlying infection. In the 1990s, researchers determined that a treatment known as activated protein C, a version of a chemical that the body produces naturally in certain circumstances, improved survival in patients who were given a diagnosis of sepsis. Activated protein C became standard treatment for years, despite the known risk of causing abnormal bleeding. When years of clinical experience were examined and analyzed however, investigators determined that activated protein C did not provide a benefit in the treatment of sepsis, and it was withdrawn as standard therapy.

All of the foregoing examples demonstrate that, even with a scientific approach, the methods adopted into modern medicine are not foolproof. There is a well-known maxim in logic that it is impossible to prove a negative, particularly that something does not exist or will not happen. There is no number of examples of an absolute proposition that cannot be undone by a single counterexample. An analogous situation applies to medicine: there is nothing that proves that what has worked for any number of previous cases will work for a particular patient, nor that a patient might not receive some benefit from an intervention that science has dismissed. Medical science is unavoidably a statistical science, because of the unmanageable number of combinations, permutations, variables and unknowns that apply to the workings of human bodies.

There is a practical limit to how scientific the practice of modern medicine can be. This results from the complexity of the human body and the overlapping clinical presentations that exist in health and illness. The clinical significance of one patient having a blood count, or hematocrit level, of 38% another of 41%, or of the same patient having similarly disparate readings three months apart is not obvious without more information. A clinical determination that something is abnormal is often simply an interpretation of statistical profiles that is more useful in comparing a particular patient to a large population than it is in proving that a particular patient has a specific disease. Moreover, it is not always obvious that the observed abnormality is causally related to the patient's complaint, or that remedying the abnormality will help and not harm the patient. A high white blood cell count can be treated, often independently of the cause, by giving medicines that prevent the body from making new white blood cells. A concerning laboratory abnormality may thus be resolved without affecting the causative pathology, and with predictably unfortunate consequences for the patient. Many concerning signs and symptoms share this characteristic, such as rapid heartbeat or respiratory rate, fever, diarrhea, and edema. Patients and their families often insist that something be done about the concerning laboratory or physical finding, without regard to how it affects the patient's underlying condition. Physicians are sometimes pressured to "treat the numbers" without regard to the clinical utility of such efforts. Physicians must distinguish between the patient's medical need for possibly risky therapy and psychological needs for reassurance and the appearance of doing something affirmative.

Popular perception often conflicts with medical reality. Patients often perceive that all diseases are readily diagnosable because of the availability of highly sophisticated diagnostic technologies such as computed tomography scanners, magnetic resonance imaging devices and sensitive genetic probes. Likewise, the ever-expanding number of cures that medical science provides can create the illusion that all diseases have a cure, if only more diligence were applied to finding them. The reality of modern medicine is, however, that sometimes diseases and injuries can be remedied, sometimes they can be accommodated and sometimes they can only be accepted, along with their inevitable consequences. Physicians and other healthcare practitioners sometimes provide care that is mostly ceremonial, for the same reasons and to the same effect as that provided by shamans centuries ago.

The progress of medicine and healthcare, as with any form of progress, allows one to observe trends and develop expectations. A reasonable interpretation of history suggests that the goal of healthcare will not be to eliminate disease or dispel the effects of trauma. Progress brings with it not only new cures and diagnostic technologies, but new diseases as well. Infections with the human immunodeficiency virus and legionella bacterium were only recognized in the past century, and the several disease states associated with obesity were unheard of by, or perhaps even inconceivable to, people more concerned with starving to death.

The progress of medical practice is generally in the direction of greater efficiency, more standardization and more focused therapies. Surgical procedures have become progressively less invasive with the desirable outcomes of fewer complications and quicker recovery times. Interventions that at one time required large, disfiguring incisions, such as removal of a gall bladder or repair of a hernia, are now accomplished with specialized instruments requiring incisions less than an inch long. Recovery periods have been shortened accordingly, allowing patients to return to a degree of normality within days rather than weeks. Complicated vascular repairs, that once involved hours of risky surgery, are now achieved with small devices passed through the patient's blood vessels. Many therapeutic alterations of body structures are now accomplished without the necessity of disassembly and reassembly. Robots are finding greater use in surgery, enabling operators to repair smaller and smaller structures and perform older procedures with greater precision. The advances in surgical techniques and technology are truly objective improvements. They hold out the promise that procedures will become more effective, less costly and applicable to a greater number of maladies.

Technology has also led to the decentralization of medical decision-making. This may not be of equal benefit in each individual case, but for health care systems as a whole it makes expertise more widely available and, in theory, at least makes accessing that expertise more efficient. Radiologists quite commonly read and interpret radiographs and other imaging studies that they are able to access from computers, regardless of the location of the patient. Thus, these physicians are able to provide services to multiple hospitals at the same time, even though they may be hundreds of miles from the patient. The same technology allows critical care physicians to monitor patient information from remote facilities and provide some consultative and management expertise without ever laying hands on the patient. These technologies are beneficial to patients being cared for in rural or remote locations, and partially obviate the need for either the patient or the physician to travel to the other's location before care is provided or received. This improves access to care and makes that care more efficient.

Scientific study has improved our understanding of many disease states, and this has allowed for improved diagnostic and therapeutic interventions. Genetic methods and monoclonal antibody techniques have improved the ability to identify pathogens and inherited diseases, potentially allowing therapy earlier in the course of illness. This has been particularly important for degenerative conditions such as rheumatoid arthritis, cancer and some forms of hepatitis. Understanding of how environmental and lifestyle factors interact to cause injury and disease gives patients a chance to affect their clinical course and minimize the burden of illness on their lives. Advances in organ transplantation and chemotherapeutics have made it possible for patients to survive some disease that only decades ago were uniformly fatal.

Most progress in medical science is built upon previous advances; the new discoveries and technologies then become the bases for further advances, making medical science an endeavor of eternal promise. An unintended consequence of this trend is that patients may be saved from one previously incurable condition to endure life with another that remains so, such as dementia or end stage kidney disease. The advances of medical science sometimes outpace our ability to appreciate the consequences, regardless of whether those consequences are physical, psychological, ethical or social.

One consequence of the scientific and technological advance of medicine is that it is impossible for one person to keep up with it all. This naturally results in practitioners focusing their expertise into narrower, more nuanced fields. Where once a specialist may have focused on diseases of a particular organ or organ system, some specialists are now experts in particular diseases of those organs. Primary care physicians once cared for patients in their offices and admitted them and followed them in the hospital when necessary. Now, there are not only physicians who specialize in hospital care, there are those that specialize in specific parts of the hospital stay, such as only performing the initial examination and writing admission orders, or only following those who have required hospitalization for an extended period. Radiologists were once the specialized providers that interpreted imaging studies. There are now those who specialize in imaging of a specific part of the body, interpret particular types of studies or who perform interventional procedures.

Specialization is necessary in modern medicine because the complexity of medical technology and advances in medical knowledge increase the learning time required to become an expert in certain areas of care. Specialists, whether they are oncologists or kidney specialists or psychiatrists or radiologists must now relearn the essentials of their practices repeatedly over the course of their careers, and those who are unable to keep up will become effectively unskilled.

Specialization is also an inherent form of optimization, since it tends to increase the efficiency with which the specialist applies his or her skill. A patient who is able to seek the expertise of a surgeon who has done 3000 carotid artery surgeries when that procedure is necessary is more likely to enjoy the benefits of acquired knowledge and experience than if he receives care from a surgeon who has done 50 carotid surgeries, with any number of other procedures unrelated to the patient's current need. Depth of experience is more beneficial than breadth in many highly sophisticated fields. It is more efficient to receive services from an expert when those services are in his field of expertise than it is from someone whose limited experience in that field is part of a portfolio of experiences. The trend toward greater degrees of specialization is simply one element of the progress of medicine, and indeed all human progress, in the direction of greater efficiency.

Guidelines and algorithms are becoming more prevalent in modern medicine, and one of the subtle reasons for this is the trend toward a greater number of conflicting interests competing for consideration in individual medical decisions. Practically any medical decision affects the interests of some party other than the patient, and guidelines are one method of observing these competing interests. Guidelines may be promulgated with the intent of reducing waste, improving efficiency and ensuring the appropriateness of care, and these are undoubtedly valid goals. Their validity derives however from the complexity of modern medicine and the dependence of the healthcare system on parties beside the patient and physician.

Another of the trends in modern healthcare is that conflicting interests extend beyond the considerations of healthcare. It is now understood that some consideration is due to the interests of medical device manufacturers, insurance companies, hospitals, nurses, patients, family members, physicians, investors, etc., but increasingly healthcare conflicts with other societal and cultural interests such as education, public safety and infrastructure. The needs of a local school district might eventually indirectly affect the decision of what treatment is best for an octogenarian's arthritis or a demented patient's kidney failure.

The confluence of individual trends has produced an overarching change in healthcare. The decentralization of decision-making, consideration of interests that used to be regarded as subordinate to the physician-patient relationship, and the ongoing search for institutional efficiency have combined to impose the methods of mass production onto medical practice. That which was once regarded as an intimate relationship between patient and provider is now recognized as a component of an industrial complex. One of the most visible effects of this phenomenon is that physicians and other healthcare providers have become employees of larger organizations, and more and more details of an individual's care are now determined by people who never see, or are even aware of the patient. The era of a talented student sacrificing and persevering through the rigors of medical school and then starting an independent practice that would grow according to reputation and skill has been overtaken by exorbitant student debt, difficulties in starting and maintaining a private practice, and the ability of large institutions and entities to insist that their interests be considered. The result is that a new physician will likely become employed by a large group practice, or a healthcare system affiliated either with hospitals or insurers. Considerations of resource utilization and efficiency are largely responsible for this change, and it has been accompanied by trade offs.

Some desirable characteristics of medical practice have been diminished in deference to systemic considerations. One such characteristic is the time that an individual provider has available to tend to the various needs of a patient. Technology and economic pressures have combined to produce a more regimented approach to diagnosis and therapy. This has come at the expense of the notion that time spent with a patient can itself be therapeutic. Patients have a need to tell their stories, even if the detail they provide is extraneous to scientific management of the culprit malady. Patients sometimes have a need to not only be examined and studied as biological specimens, but to be understood as people with a story and a life that is impacted by the state of their health.

Changes in the nature of healthcare, even the ones that are undesirable, are for the most part rational. There are parts of the modern healthcare system that are susceptible to exploitation, and the intensely economic nature of modern medicine attracts the participation of those whose interests do not include the altruism classically associated with caring for the sick. This result, though perhaps lamentable with reference to compassion, caring, empathy and other virtues associated with medicine, is not surprising.

Modern medicine is guided to a large degree by advances in medical knowledge. More accurate and exact diagnostic methods and more precise treatment methods make the modern practice of medicine appear more deterministic. Arcane and mysterious therapies that ameliorated symptoms of various conditions have been supplanted by definitive treatments and cures provided by scientific investigation and improved understanding of disease mechanisms. This has led to the inaccurate impression that medicine has become less of an art, and more of a trade; that having an intuitive feel for what is behind a patient's complaints has been replaced by infallible diagnostic and treatment science. In some cases this is justified, as when a young person with no other known health problems feels an abnormal mass that can be biopsied, studied under a microscope and confidently determined to be benign or malignant. In other cases, the results of even the most advanced diagnostic methods are themselves only fragments of data that must be interpreted in context. Furthermore, a patient may have a pathologic condition that is amenable to advanced diagnostic methods, but this does not ensure that the patient does not also have another, more occult process that accounts for his or her distress. Modern science often makes logical fallacies seem more inviting, particularly where diagnostic studies are so sensitive that they are likely to detect some abnormality, even if it is unrelated to the condition under investigation. Correlation does not, after all, equal causation, but a significant portion of medical history involves the analysis of empirical observation and the search for correlation. Modern trends and technologies have not eliminated this process.

Even though modern science has made seemingly miraculous advances in diagnostic and treatment methods, patients still seek out the care of healthcare practitioners for problems that either may not have a definitive diagnostic test, or even if the disease is properly identified, may not have a treatment. Part of the art of medicine is making the patient feel better, and encouraging a meaningful life even when the disease is an irresistible force with an inevitable outcome. Not all diseases have a cure, or even a name, and not all cures leave the patient better off. Treating diseases and injuries can be something of an abstraction, and there may be many reasons why a physician provides a particular therapy. Sometimes treatment for physical conditions is given for psychological reasons, and vice versa. Treatments with little chance of working are given for religious or philosophical reasons, and sometimes they are given because no one knows what else to do. Science can take medical diagnosis and treatment a long way, but it will never supplant the human element. There is much about human life that is meaningful, and unrelated to the investigations of science.

Improved diagnostic methods have changed our perceptions of how common certain diseases are, and have provoked new anxieties. Some diseases that were thought of as exotic and too rare to warrant alarm appear epidemic when it becomes easier to diagnose them. In addition, risk factors for particular diseases are often treated as diseases themselves, such as abnormal cholesterol. Markers of disease are also treated as though they were separate disease states, such as abnormal liver enzymes or edema, and without the discretion and expertise of medical professionals, these markers may be normalized in a manner that is much to the patient's disadvantage.

The growth of healthcare as a policy discipline has altered the intimate relationship between a patient and an individual provider. Considerations that at one time would have been ignored in favor of the patient's interests are now given at least some deference. The intrusion of policy and institutional complexity into individual medical considerations also gives rise to a disquieting conundrum. A physician's ability to provide treatment for a patient suffering from a particular condition may depend on how that condition is regarded by policy makers or perceived by society. The ability to treat certain conditions may depend on the resources available to make such treatment a societal priority, with the inevitable consequence that some diseases will be treated more favorably than others, for no other reason than better marketing.

In many ways the modern practice of medicine is the same as it has been for centuries: a relationship between a patient and a practitioner who uses knowledge, experience and judgment to make decisions in the interests of the patient's better health. Science, innovation, economics, politics and the natural forces that determine the behavior of aging bureaucracies and institutions will inevitably make some things better and some things worse.

8

ATROPOS
THE END

There is something of a paradox in the notion that things as common and universal as disease and injury are regarded as abnormal. The typical experience of disease, such as with the common cold or influenza, as something unwelcome is readily distinguished from the presumed "normal" state of good health. The observation that the common cold is common seems not to matter, and the natural tendency is to regard the transient state as an anomaly. The perception of disease and injury as irregular arises not only because they are noted to be deviations from the norm, but also because they are deviations from the desirable. The fact that many common maladies and injuries are transient and leave no lasting effects makes it easy to reject them as having little or no enduring significance.

Transient conditions are only a subset of the possible afflictions that may befall a person. Some diseases are chronic, requiring alterations in lifestyle and habits; others are disabling or associated with continuing misery; and others are reliably fatal. Sometimes a disease or injury assumes such prominence in a person's life that he or she adopts them as part of an identity, self-describing as "a diabetic," "a paraplegic," or a "breast cancer survivor."

Individual diseases and injuries may be objectively abnormal, but experiencing them or suffering with them is not. Few people make it from one end of life to the other without encountering them. The process of dealing with significant diseases and injuries can consume a great deal of a person's time, energy and resilience, and sometimes health issues become a defining part of a person's life.

The impression of medicine that one gets as a patient is different from that which results from other perspectives. A person's experience with a significant disease or injury can be quite personal, and the benefit of modern medicine will vary accordingly. People respond differently to diagnoses of cancer, a stroke, or injury requiring amputation. People have different expectations of healthcare, some rational and others not, even at times foregoing potential cures of disease because of conflicts with other values. It is tempting to assume that there is an obvious and objective ranking of priorities that determine how people will behave when confronted with a health issue. Common sense appears to suggest that people will prefer lifestyle changes to increased risk of illness, or loss of independence to the risk of a potentially fatal event. In reality however, disease and ominous diagnoses affect more than just biological descriptions of a person's health. A particular diagnosis may affect that person's self-image, relationship with loved ones and lifelong ambitions. The loss of autonomy and independence that some forms of medical therapy entail may be a price greater than some people are willing to pay. Modern medicine may offer some people the prospect of cures, reduced burdens of disease and better quality of life than was available to previous generations afflicted with the same maladies; yet the same therapies may appear to others as unwanted intrusions or provide marginal benefits that do not justify the trouble.

No one can prescribe how an individual patient should view a particular disease. Some people respond to a given diagnosis with disappointment; others with anger, fear or denial. Some patients are more concerned with how their illness will affect family members, and others will wonder if a serious disease has any meaning for their life beyond ill health. Even when the diagnosis is terminal and the prognosis grim, patients will vary in their perception of life, disease and the role of medicine. Some people will want to go out kicking and screaming, "raging against the dying of the light" in Dylan Thomas's poetic phrase. Others accept the inevitable with quiet resignation.

Sometimes the most difficult thing associated with an ominous diagnosis is the burden on the patient to decide how he or she wants to live the rest of their lives. The choices often present jarring contrasts: living on a hospital ward, getting poked, prodded, sampled, and infused in an all-out attempt to face down a nefarious foe, or to accept the natural course but postpone the influence of disease to the end, and live on one's own terms, if only for a short while.

Just as people's impression of injury and disease tends to be personal, so too do expectations of healthcare. Some people seek out diagnosis and therapy as something of a formality, to assure themselves that they did everything possible to forestall the inevitable, even if they had little expectation of benefit. Others just want something to ease the journey, and yet others have the same expectation of modern medicine that people in previous centuries had of magic. While it is tempting for physicians and other healthcare providers to assume that patients merely want treatment to cure an illness, heal an injury or forestall death, patients' priorities may differ. Some patients who are wracked with pain will only want the pain relieved, regardless of any other side effects. Others may be willing to endure some discomfort to remain mentally alert and to spend their time fully aware of each moment with their loved ones.

Patient's demands are sometimes at cross-purposes with each other. Denial and a need to retain a sense of control may complicate what is otherwise standard therapy; it does not do any good to refuse interventions when they might be beneficial only to demand them when they are futile. Illness is sometimes a very prominent part of a person's life, and not everyone knows in advance what parts of life are most meaningful. Perhaps someone who is given a diagnosis of terminal cancer will decide that earlier interests are no longer as important.

Patients have idiosyncratic responses not only to the substance of unfavorable news, but to the form as well. A practitioner can never be quite certain what specific phrase or word choice will resonate with a patient, and therefore cannot afford unguarded or trite embellishment. When a surgeon counsels a cancer patient about the five-year survival associated with his diagnosis, it is possible that the patient does not appreciate the specific data in percentages nearly as much as discussing the possibility that he will be dead of cancer in five years.

People have different approaches to dealing with disease. Some people view illness as an adversary to be conquered, others as a predator to be avoided. Some people will want to feel that they are in control of the campaign to vanquish the pathologic enemy; others will simply want to be cared for and relinquish all responsibility for their health to others. Some people view struggle with disease as a meaningful and clarifying part of life, others regard it as a spoiler, an unwelcome obstacle to long-cherished goals and beliefs.

Patients' views and expectations of their healthcare also change when confronted with stark and sobering reports that their heath is in headlong retreat, that the inevitable is now the imminent. Some patients and their families expect miracles, some expect explanations and some expect recourse. Medicine however, like all human institutions has limits; there are some things that it cannot provide and there are some expectations it cannot meet.

The reality that medicine has limits is not altered by perspective. Medicine is powerless when applied to a body that has been spent. In order for medicine to have a practical effect the body must retain enough of a reserve to participate in recovery. As the body ages both the rate and the absolute amount of this recovery declines until the descent of health is unstoppable. For a while, most people have some capacity to compensate for this deterioration, creating the illusion that health is being maintained, and luring both the hopeful and the worried into the illusion that things are simply going on as before. The ability to compensate for subtle losses of health can be quite robust, and octogenarians, nonagenarians and centenarians can remain remarkably "sharp" and active even as their limits are strained and the inevitable proceeds. Healthcare and medicine can be useful in this process, even as it is unable to stop it.

Nearly all medicine is a form of jury-rigging, the product of ingenuity and resourcefulness. Medicine is not part of mankind's natural endowment. The biology of the human body did not develop in anticipation that potions and elixirs would modify its natural functions, or that it would be cut open in pursuit of improved health. The processes that the body uses to recover from surgery are those our ancestors used to recover from being mauled by animals. The beneficial effects of medicine are partly due to human design, are sometimes accidental, and nearly always owe much to the human body's resilience and ability to heal.

When the disease has progressed beyond the body's ability to recover, the scientific aspect of medicine yields diminishing returns. Patients and their families will often not accept this fact, and respond to deteriorating health with more forceful demands for diagnosis, resort to exotic therapies, and referral to anonymous experts. A peculiar aspect of advanced technological societies is reluctance to acknowledge that technology can't solve every problem, and emotional demands will not produce therapies where there otherwise are none. Anger, stubbornness, and determination do not make otherwise futile interventions effective. This becomes increasingly frustrating for patients and families as standard interventions become less and less effective and the adverse effects become more alarming. The difference between interventions that produce desirable and undesirable effects becomes smaller and smaller until medical therapies do as much harm as good. These scenarios do provide some useful prognostic clues however. If the difference between a patient living or dying depends on whether he gets 40 milligrams of some medicine instead of 50, the patient is very likely to die regardless.

One ritual of disease and injury that seems to have persisted throughout history is that of the vigil; the anxious wait for the crisis to pass or the patient to succumb. The somber watch at the patient's bedside is one of the more human experiences, and quite possibly one of the more meaningful ones, that will likely never be made obsolete. Modern technology may alter some of the details but the essence remains the same. One of the things that advanced monitoring methods provides is a stream of data that patients and loved ones use to infer, from moment to moment, the patient's course. Family members sometimes stare for hours on end at heart monitors and oxygen saturation meters; they inquire daily about laboratory studies that reflect the patient's kidney or liver function; they want steady reports of urine output and blood pressure readings. Serious disease is often a great unknown, and people who are accustomed to ordering their lives around timely information avidly seek any clue to the impending outcome.

Sometimes the information is misleading. There is a reason why no major league baseball teams completes a season undefeated, and that is that everyone has good days and bad days. It is tempting to get overly optimistic on the good days and to sink into despair on the bad days, but these are intrinsic to daily life in both sickness and health. The challenge is to get neither too optimistic nor too morose over the natural fluctuations that accompany serious diseases and injuries. The reality of many diseases however is that a point is reached where the overall trend toward improvement is no longer realistic, and subsequent days are expected to be worse than those that preceded them. Sometimes the really important decisions in life are made for us. The moment that this point is reached is usually subtle, recognized only in retrospect. The dawning realization is often difficult for patients and their families, but is also frequently accompanied by a sense of relief, a clarifying portent that implies both opportunity and finality.

The role and value of medicine change when a disease is terminal. The drama and pathos of terminal illness often obscures the possibility that people are capable of being happy while they are dying. This possibility creates a role for medicine even when the goal of cure, or even a temporary reprieve, is beyond reach. Healthcare providers of all disciplines and methods can provide comfort, information and, above all, a human interaction that bridges the experience of mysterious technologies, chemicals and sterile rituals with that of a universal human reality. Healthcare varies in its methods and philosophies, in its promises and pretensions. It sometimes claims the credit that properly belongs to good fortune and assigns its own blame elsewhere. Sometimes the patient derives some good from it, sometimes not, but the variety of healthcare tends to assume the same form at the end of the patient's life: that of human beings, through reason and experience and compassion trying to ensure that the final stages of a person's life are not meaningless biological formalities.

Healthcare and medicine have a place even when they can no longer improve physical health.

Healthcare endures as a human institution, not only because of its near miraculous successes in treating disease and injury, but because of what it has to offer in the face of that ultimate human reality with which this book began: everybody dies.

BIBLIOGRAPHY

Adler M. *The Great Ideas: A Syntopicon*. Chicago: Encyclopedia Britannica; 1952

Bartlett J, ed. *Familiar Quotations*, 15th ed. Boston: Little, Brown and Co. ; 1980

Chadwick B. *George Washington's War*. Naperville Ill.: Sourcebooks; 2004

Fagothey A. *Right and Reason: Ethics in theory and practice*, 6th ed. St. Louis: Mosby; 1976

Gilman AG, Rall TW, Nies AS, Taylor P, eds. *Goodman & Gilman's The Pharmacological Basis of Therapeutics*, 8th ed. New York: Pergamon; 1990

Hawking S. *A Brief History of Time*. New York: Bantam Books; 1996

Hippocrates. *Of the Epidemics*. accessed at classics.mit.edu/Hippocrates/Epidemics.html

Lifton RJ. *The Nazi Doctors: Medical killing and the psychology of genocide*. Basic Books; 1986.

Markel H. *Becoming a physician: "I swear by Apollo" – On taking the Hippocratic Oath*. N Engl J Med, 350:2026 (2004).

McCullough D. *1776*. New York: Simon & Schuster; 2005

Plato. *Laws*. Accessed at classics.mit.edu/Plato.laws.html

Rose BD. *Clinical Physiology of Acid-Base and Electrolyte Disorders*, 3rd ed. New York: McGraw Hill; 1989

South Tyrol Museum of Archeology. *Ötzi-the Iceman.* www.iceman.it/en/node/260

U. S. Food and Drug Administration. FDA Drug Safety Communication: Voluntary market withdrawal of Xigris [drotrecogin alfa (activated)] due to failure to show a survival benefit. 10/25/2011.
www.fda.gov/Drugs/DrugSafety/ucm277114.htm

Witters LA. *The blooming of the French lilac*. Journal of Clinical Investigation, 108:1105-1107, (October, 2001).

ABOUT THE AUTHOR

Joseph Batuello is a physician practicing hospital medicine in Aurora, Colorado. He is author of *End of Life Decisions: A practical guide.*

www.ingramcontent.com/pod-product-compliance
Lightning Source LLC
Chambersburg PA
CBHW030934180526
45163CB00002B/560